Digital Health Care in Taiwan

Po-Chang Lee • Joyce Tsung-Hsi Wang
Tzu-Yu Chen • Chia-Hui Peng
Editors

Digital Health Care in Taiwan

Innovations of National Health Insurance

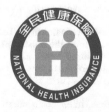

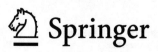

Editors
Po-Chang Lee
National Health Insurance Administration
Ministry of Health and Welfare, Taiwan
Taipei, Taiwan

Joyce Tsung-Hsi Wang
National Health Insurance Administration
Ministry of Health and Welfare, Taiwan
Taipei, Taiwan

Tzu-Yu Chen
National Health Insurance Administration
Ministry of Health and Welfare, Taiwan
Taipei, Taiwan

Chia-Hui Peng
National Health Insurance Administration
Ministry of Health and Welfare, Taiwan
Taipei, Taiwan

ISBN 978-3-031-05162-3   ISBN 978-3-031-05160-9   (eBook)
https://doi.org/10.1007/978-3-031-05160-9

This Springer imprint is published by the registered company Springer Nature Switzerland AG
The registered company address is: Gewerbestrasse 11, 6330 Cham, Switzerland

Foreword

Investing in the National Health Insurance Is Investing in Health

The *Reform Diary 2.0* published by the National Health Insurance Administration (NHIA) in May 2021 has attracted attention from the medical sector and the general public. It was a wonderful channel for readers to understand the reforms that the NHIA has made in the past few years and the improvements that it plans to make. Now, the newly released *Digital Health Care in Taiwan: Innovations of National Health Insurance* introduces the operation of the National Health Insurance (NHI) and how Taiwan utilises information and communication technology to improve health care in detail.

In Taiwan, because of universal healthcare coverage, citizens can enjoy high accessibility and quality health care as the strongest backing for preventing and controlling pandemic outbreaks. All confirmed COVID-19 cases in Taiwan can obtain comprehensive medical care provided by dedicated healthcare providers and covered by the national budget. Therefore, the pandemic was fairly effectively controlled. However, owing to the advancement of medical technology and the ageing population, the annual expenditures of the NHI have been constantly higher than the growth of income. The safety reserve accumulated in the past few years will not be enough to cover the deficits in the future. Therefore, under the National Health Insurance's principle of income–expenditure linkage, the Executive Yuan approved the Ministry of Health and Welfare's proposal to adjust the premium rate for the NHI from 4.69% to 5.17% at the end of 2020. It is hoped that by cross-sharing the financial burden, we can stabilise the funding of the National Health Insurance and continue to provide high-quality medical services. The National Health Insurance was made possible by contributions from all nationals, and it has become the strongest backing for everyone in Taiwan.

However, to maintain the sustainability of the NHI, in addition to balancing income and expenditure, we have to update its systems and relevant measures to keep pace with modern trends. The NHIA should review policies that reduce unnecessary medical services, promote fair burden and improve the quality of care. Necessary measures and reform plans have been initiated to strengthen these efforts. Among them are the rights and responsibilities of citizens travelling overseas, fair calculation of the supplementary premium and the co-payment of medical costs. Moreover, the NHIA should reduce waste by integrating medical resources for effective utilisation, sharing medical information through the NHI MediCloud system and suppressing improper consumption of medical resources. In addition, a 4- to 6-year long- to mid-term reform plan should be implemented to reform the health insurance coverage, as well as payment and healthcare systems. It is aimed to integrate the public health system and resources from the NHI to comprehensively improve the quality of medical care for all citizens.

Article 1 of the National Health Insurance Law declares clearly that the NHI was enacted to promote the health of all nationals. Therefore, improving the health of every individual in Taiwan is its ultimate goal . As the statutory insurer of the NHI, the NHIA shoulders heavy responsibilities to achieve this goal. It is hoped that through the publication of this book, the public can have a better understanding of the purpose of the NHI. Furthermore, it is hoped that through the efforts of the NHIA, all nationals can realise that investing in the NHI is an investment in health. With support from all sectors of society for the NHI, we can work together to build a sustainable healthcare system that benefits all people. Finally, for the NHIA, the burden is heavy and the road is long.

Shih-Chung Chen, D.D.S.
Minister of Health and Welfare,
Taiwan
Taipei, Taiwan

Preface

Thoughts on Reforming the National Health Insurance

During the past 3 years, the National Health Insurance Administration (NHIA) has published two books, *National Health Insurance Reform Diary 1.0* and *National Health Insurance Reform Diary 2.0*. We now honorably present *Digital Health Care in Taiwan: Innovations of National Health Insurance*, a tangible result of the NHIA welcoming more than 500 global visitors each year to exchange health-related policies and implementation struggles. By publishing this book, we hope to offer a better understanding of the healthcare system in Taiwan to officials at health departments worldwide. The following figure depicts the reform framework using National Health Insurance (NHI) core values.

Reduce misuse	• Enhance efficiency by integrating resources • Share data through the NHI MediCloud system • Reduce misuse of medical resources
Adjust beneficiary qualification	• Revise rights and obligations of citizens based overseas • Adjust basement of supplementary premium • Modify copayment regulation
Improve quality	• 4~6 years "NHI mid/long-term development plan" • Reform NHI reimbursement and payment policy • Integrate public health system and NHI resources

Reform consistent with NHI core values

As the Director General of the NHIA, I have been thinking a lot about the expense increases we negotiate with the medical profession every year. Each relative value unit (RVU) never equals New Taiwan dollar (NTD) 1, and the medical profession has always been quite unpleased by the relatively flat growth in medical payments. However, the fundamental problem of increasing RVUs is the number of medical visits. For example, Western medicine medical visits have grown by nearly six million visits per year. As long as medical visits do not decrease, the "sweat hospital" issue (discussed later) will remain unsolved. However, for hospitals, more medical visits mean a greater chance to provide self-paid medical services. Looking through financial reports from hospitals with 2018 revenues of more than NTD 200 million reveals that 23.48% of their revenue comes from registration fees and self-payments. For clinics, a major revenue source is registration fees not covered by the NHI. Therefore, reducing medical visits is a difficult problem not only because of public behavior but also because of doctors' mindsets, which can be even tougher to deal with.

The core of this improvement plan is the promotion of "rising co-payment." I believe that increased co-payments can change the behavior of both patients and doctors. The number of those who have thoughts of "hospital shopping" will be expected to drop, leading to fewer medical visits. Subsequently, the value of the RVU will grow, and medical professionals will be able to earn more reasonable pay from the same effort.

The second highlight of my improvement plan is the "digital transformation of the healthcare system." The NHI MediCloud System was originally built to share individuals' medication and examination reports, and this system received high praise from the medical profession. Both the NHI MediCloud System and the "NHI card" played important roles in providing information about "TOCC" (travel, occupation, cluster, and contact) and the "Name-Based Medical Mask Distribution System" in the battle against COVID-19 in 2020.

With technological developments and innovation breakthroughs, a wave of artificial intelligence (AI) has swept the world. The most noteworthy of these in medicine has been using big data and medical images from the NHI system to stimulate AI application development and transform care services for disease. Various innovations and applications have been incubated concurrently with the development of the NHI database and "My Health Bank," further fostering healthcare and medical solutions that benefit all people in Taiwan.

I would like to mention "telemedicine" in particular. Taiwan's strong, solid information technology industry creates a smart telemedicine model through information and communication network technology, so medical care is no longer limited by distance. In addition, "home-based medical care" is a new medical trend in which we encourage medical professionals to participate in teams. With new technology, we advance the "NHI card" to the "virtual NHI card" and apply for "home-based medical care." I hope to establish a new era of the NHI medical service model as soon as possible.

The third key point of my reform plan is "leading medical care to a new economic model." Driven by advancements in cancer treatment, the proper use of optimal medication through precision medicine in oncology has become a trend. Compared with traditional medical care, when undergoing targeted therapy and immunotherapy, patients are treated with the most effective medicine according to their individual biomarkers to achieve the goal of "prescribing the right medicine." This eliminates the cost of ineffective medication and also reduces the risk of patient side effects. Because of the inseparable relationship between NHI and medical care, the introduction of new medicines, medical devices, and medical technologies into the system also indirectly helps Taiwan's biotechnology and medicine industry find its own path.

The final point of my reform plan focuses on the "outdated NHI fee schedule and system." Medical technology and equipment have made great progress over the past two decades, and patients' clinical conditions have become more complicated. The human and material resources invested in treatment are relatively greater and more professional. Therefore, we must deal with the outdated NHI fee schedule and system more pragmatically. In addition to responding to the contributions of medical professionals, we must facilitate the balanced development of the medical system. We will continue to review the reasonableness of the NHI fee schedule and provide the public with high-quality medical services.

I started as a surgery professor, then became a hospital director, and now I am Director General of the NHIA. I have seen changes that need to be made in the NHI system. But it takes time to improve. After all, procedures must be followed to ensure effective and lasting systematic reform. I take my job seriously, planning out blueprints and implementing policies. My colleagues and I at the NHIA will actively work with partners in the medical profession to do our part for the people. This book includes many insights and a reformation focus, and we welcome all kinds of advice for further improvements.

Taipei, Taiwan   Po-Chang Lee, M.D., M.T.L.

Acknowledgments

First, I especially wish to thank President Tsai Ing-wen, Vice President Lai Ching-Te, Former Vice President Chen Jian-Ren, Senior Advisor to the President Li Ming-Liang, Minister of Ministry of Health and Welfare Chen Shih-Chung, and Former Minister of Health and Welfare Lin Zou-Yan, who appointed me to be the Director General of the National Health Insurance Administration, which I am honored to be a part of. Thank you for letting me serve and continue the reform project of the National Health Insurance.

This book is part of the 2021 Technology Development Project—Provision of Sustainable Quality Healthcare, funded by the Ministry of Health and Welfare, Taiwan.

I extend my gratitude to my brother, Dr. Lee Po-Huang, who has been extremely supportive throughout my career.

I would like to thank the dedicated reviewers, whose feedback and commentary have helped me immensely. I would also like to thank my peers and team at the National Health Insurance Administration—without the experiences and support I have received from them, this book would not be published.

Information Management Division:
Kuo-Lung Lee, Hau-Chuen Sun, Mei-Chu Wang, Chi-Shun Chen, Chun-Yu Pang, Hsiu-Lan Chen, Shu-Ling Huang, Ruey-yuh Duh, Tzu-Yu Chen, Shun-Liang Tang, Hui-Ping Weng, Yi-Ming Ho, Zi-Fang Chen

Medical Affairs Division:
Chia-Pin Wu, Tso-Chen Chang, Pei-Shuan Han, Hsiu-Wen Yang, Yi-Chieh Chen, Tsui-Chen Tsai, Li-Li Liu, Yu-Chi Hung, Lin-Yi Liu, Chin-Mei Lin, Yu-Ying Huang, Yu-Chen Yang, Chia-Pei Teng, Yu-Fen Chang, Tzu-Yen Lu, You-Jun Lin, Yu-Fen Lin, Chang-Chi Wei, You-Jun Lin, Huey-Jen You

Financial Analysis Division:
Yi-Lin Lai, Hsiao-Chuan Yang, Ya-Huei Yang, Huang-Chen Chang

Enrollment Division:
Chien-Chiang Huang, Chien-Hui Yu, Jen-Hui Lee, Pei-Chun Hsish, Jia-Rou Ferng

Medical Review and Pharmaceutical Benefits Division:
Ming-Tzu Hsu, Yu-Fen Lin, Hao-Hsuan Kao, Ruby Yu-Wen Huang, Hui-Ping Chang, Heng-Jung Lien, Yi-Chieh Lin, Hui-Wen Lo, Shih-Ting Liu, Chang-Jr Chen, Ruo-Han Yeh, Hsiao-Feng Ho, Yu-Neng Lin, Shu-Ya Chang, Chu-Chun Tu, Chi-Chang Lin, Shu-Lien Chien, Ju-Hsun Chang, Wen-Fuh Tseng, Yin-Ting Pan, Shu-Yi Chen, Chiung-Hsuan Huang, Ya-An Tsai, Pei-Shin Lo

Press Room:
Chien Fu Chan

Taipei Division:
Ming Hsin Liao, Pei-Chi Wang, Tsuey-Lan Moh, Pao-Fong Lin, Jong-Yih Sheu

Planning Division:
Wei-Ying Chen, Wei- Siang Jhao, Pi-Yun Sun, Chen-Yin Kuo, Shin-Yi Chuang, Yen-Hsiu Liu, Yuan-Ting Tsai, Wei-Lun Lo, You-Xin Liao Chia-Hui Peng

Kaoping Division:
Hui-Ting Hsieh

Ministry of Health and Welfare:
Fu-Chung Wang, Lin-Chih Chang

Finally, I would like to dedicate this book to all the healthcare professionals in Taiwan, safeguarding the health and well-being of the island's 23 million citizens.

Po-Chang Lee, M.D., M.T.L.

Contents

About the Contributors

Wen-Wen Chang, M.S. has served as a government official in Taiwan after graduating from the Department of Insurance of Feng Chia University in 1988. She also earned a master's degree in 2006 from the Institute of Medical Management of Chang Gung University. In the beginning, she served in the Department of Medical Affairs in the Bureau of Labor Insurance from 1989 to 1994. She has been planning and implementing the NHI in Taiwan for more than 27 years. Since 1994, she has been responsible for planning and building the medical claims system in the NHI Preparation Office. After the implementation of NHI, she was in charge of medical claims in outpatient settings. As one of the section chiefs in the Medical Affairs Division (MAD), she pushed forward the Global Budget (GB) System Program in 2002. During 16 years of service, she participated in GB negotiation, and she also assisted in dealing with several urgent events. She managed the hospital financial crisis due to SARS in 2003, and she monitored and succored the 627 dust explosion victims. In 2018, she left MAD for the Financial Analysis Division to oversee the planning of financial sustainability. She was assigned to the National Health Insurance Administration Northern Division and served as deputy director in 2019. Then, she was promoted to director in 2020. Wen-Wen not only transferred from planning to first-line execution but also became a leader and will dedicate herself to achieving the goal of helping people to "live longer, better and healthier lives" in the future.

Yu-Hsuan Chang, B.A., M.A., M.S., Ph.D. is the counselor of the Ministry of Health and Welfare and the director of the office of Congressional Liaison. She is responsible for communication between the Ministry and the Legislative Yuan to assist the passage of relevant bills and budget in the Congress. She is also an assistant professor at National Taipei University of Nursing and Health Sciences. She graduated from the College of Law at National Taiwan University, and holds three master's degrees from National Taiwan University in the Institute of Health Policy & Management, the Institute of Political Science, and the Institute of Library and Information Management respectively, as well as a Ph.D. from National Taiwan Normal University. She has been serving in the field of health management in the public sector since 1994. She has been engaged in the revision of the health insurance law since she served as the section chief of Legal Affairs of the NHIA. She has more than 25 years of practical experience in the NHI and has served as the director of the Planning Division of the NHIA since 2013. She is committed to the application and discussion of NHI big data. She focuses on multiple health and welfare areas, such as Taiwan's COVID-19 epidemic prevention work, long-term care services, national health promotion, public hygiene, mental wellness, and social security affairs.

Yu-Pin Chang, M.P.H. is the director of the Medical Affairs Division of the NHIA, and oversees the implementation of the reimbursement and payment scheme and related policies of Taiwan's NHI system. 93% of Taiwan's medical and healthcare institutions are covered by this system. Director Chang has worked at NHIA for more than 20 years. He is one of the initial designers for developing the health insurance Integrated Circuit (IC) card system. More than 99% of residents, accounting for over 23 million health insurance IC cards, have been distributed in Taiwan. Health data are uploaded to the NHIA database nationwide through the IC card. The health database has become one of the largest in the world.Director Chang has extensive experience in the health sector, specializing in public health, digital health, and medical tourism. Before joining the NHIA, he served as section chief in the Department of Medical Affairs of the Ministry of Health and Welfare from 2014 to 2017. He earned his MPH degree at National Yang-Ming University and bachelor's degree in public health at China Medical University.

Mei-Hsin Chen, L.L.M. holds a master's degree in law from National Chengchi University. She is currently the director of the Financial Analysis Division, NHIA, Ministry of Health and Welfare. She has worked in the NHIA since the launch of the NHI in 1995 and worked as section chief of the Legal Affairs Section, Planning Division, senior executive officer of the Planning Division, and deputy director of the Financial Analysis Division.

Shu-Ching Chiang, B.S. holds a bachelor's degree in insurance from Tamkang University. She is currently the director of the Enrollment Division, NHIA, Ministry of Health and Welfare, and previously worked as deputy director and senior executive officer of the Enrollment Division, chief of Taipei Division, NHIA, Ministry of Health and Welfare. Her expertise focuses on NHI enrollment regulation and policy, premium collection planning, the NHI card and enrollment data management, and enrollment-relevant research and analysis. Based on a solid foundation in the field of enrollment for over 20 years, she is dedicated to improving the equality of enrollment policy and refining the reasonableness of the enrollment operation of the NHI.

Chih-Hsing Ho, L.L.M., J.S.M., Ph.D. is an Associate Research Fellow/Associate Professor at the Institute of European and American Studies, and the Research Center for Information Technology Innovation (joint appointment), Academia

Sinica, Taiwan. Her research focuses on the nexus of law and medicine in general, with particular attention to the governance of genomics and newly emerging technologies, such as biobanks, big data, and artificial intelligence (AI). She serves as a Member of the NHIA's Legal Advisory and AI Data Access Committees. She has also been appointed to the Taiwan Ministry of Health and Welfare's Biobank Ethics and Governance Council, and the Consultation and Review Board at the National Biobank Consortium of Taiwan. She holds a Ph.D. in law from the London School of Economics, where she was an Olive Stone Scholar and an awardee of the Morris Finer Memorial Scholarship. She obtained her first law degree from Taiwan and later received her LLM from Columbia Law School and a JSM from Stanford Law School. Before moving back to Taipei in 2014, she worked at the Centre for Medical Ethics and Law at the University of Hong Kong. Her works appear in many renowned international journals, such as *Nature Genetics*, *BMC Medical Ethics*, *Computer Law & Security Review*, and *Medical Law International*. Since 2016, she has served as an Associate Editor for ELSI in Science and Genetics-Frontiers.

Chun-Fu Lee, M.S. has been the director of the Central Division of the NHIA, Ministry of Health and Welfare from October 2020 to the present. Before this, director Lee served as director of the Medical Affairs Division (MAD) from September 2017 to October 2020. She was Senior Executive Officer in the Taipei division of the NHIA from January 2016 to September 2017. In January 2005, she became the section director of payment schemes in the MAD, Bureau of National Health Insurance (now NHIA). She adopted the NHI payment system (e.g., TW-DRGS, Capitation, GB, ICD-10-CM/PCS coding system). She was promoted to Senior Executive Officer in March 2011 and served as deputy director in January 2014. From 2002 through 2005, she served as the director of Medical Administration in Taipei Municipal Hospital. In this position, she led efforts to develop a health information system for hospital management. From 1994 through 2000, she served as the staff of the Performance Management Section in Taipei Veteran General Hospital, where she designed an indicator to monitor hospital performance. From 1991 through 1994, she served as the Department of Labor Insurance staff, Council of Labor Affairs Executive Yuan, setting the fee schedule that the labor insurance pays the provider. She graduated from Yang-Ming Medical University with a master's degree in Health Administration in 1991.

Min-Yu Lee, M.P.A. graduated from Tunghai University in Taichung and earned a master's degree in public administration from National Dong Hwa University in Hualien County. She has been the director of the Eastern Division of NHIA Ministry of Health and Welfare since March 2010. Since the Bureau was launched in 1995, she has been an employee of the Eastern Brunch for more than 27 years. She is familiar with the work and has accumulated rich work experience. She is enthusiastic about serving insured units and cares about the quality of health care around Hualien and Taitung County.

Po-Chang Lee, M.D., M.T.L. has served as a surgeon and professor in the Taoyuan Provincial Hospital and National Cheng Kung University Hospital after graduating from the Department of Medicine of Taipei Medical College in 1979. He has been involved in the clinical and research fields of organ transplantation for more than 40 years. He has received teacher honors many times and has assisted more than a thousand patients receiving kidney transplants.In 2011, he took over as the chairman of the Taiwan Organ Registry and Sharing Center. During his term as chairman, he was dedicated to promoting the paired exchange of living donor kidney transplantation between nonrelatives, and prioritizing the third-degree relatives and spouses of organ donors in the waiting list. As a result of his enthusiastic promotion, the concept of "willingness to share" took root in people's hearts, and the number of domestic donors has reached new heights.Since May 2016, when he took over the position as the Director General of the NHIA, he has integrated his medical and legal expertise to implement various NHI system reforms, including promoting a named dual-review system to reduce disparity; safeguarding vulnerable people and unlocking the link between owing arrears and medical treatment; gradually relaxing payment conditions for new all-oral drugs to implement the hepatitis C eradication policy; promoting a tiered medical care system and implementation of two-way referral; improving "NHI MediCloud System" and allowing "My Health Bank" to be combined with the health management industry, NHI database, and AI applications, which made outstanding contributions to Taiwan's digital healthcare development. In August 2019, the "APEC Conference on Enhancing Medical and Disease Management" was hosted. About 40 people from 13 economies and foreign guests were invited to Taiwan. The event was unprecedented and greatly improved the visibility of universal health insurance in the international community. During his term as Director General of the NHIA, he made great contributions to the perseverance and system improvement of the NHI system. The public's satisfaction with the NHI increased from 81.7% in 2016 to 90.2% in 2020, hitting record highs, making the NHI one of the most popular public policies.

Chun-Mei Lin, Ph.D. is a senior director at the NHIA. She has a PhD degree in information and industrial management at National Cheng Kung University. She has over 20 years of experience in health insurance management. Her main responsibilities are to control southern region health expenditure within the annual budget, to analyze variation in clinical practice and delivery of healthcare services to improve quality of care, and to integrate the research findings concerning the knowledge procurement from claims data and practice, particularly healthcare fraud detection via data mining and information disclosures.

Shu-Hwa Lin, M.P.H. is director of NHIA-Kaoping Division, Ministry of Health and Welfare. She holds a master's degree in public health from National Taiwan University in Taipei, Taiwan. Before taking a job at the NHIA, Ms. Lin served as a supervisor at the Kaohsiung Municipal Min-Sheng Hospital, dedicated to medical record management, information system development, and medical management-related businesses. Ms. Lin has been working for the National Health Insurance Department since the establishment of the Bureau of National Health Insurance in 1995 and has experienced various positions during that period. It is worth mentioning that during her tenure as the director of the NHIA-Southern Division, she supervised the relevant emergency response operations after the Tainan earthquake in 2016 with outstanding performance. Now, she will continue to contribute her knowledge and pass on her years of work experience to the younger generation.

Yu-Chuan Liu, M.P.H. holds a master's degree in Institute of Health Policy and Management from National Taiwan University. She is currently the director of the NHIA-Taipei Division. Before this, director Liu served as deputy head of the MAD and the Taipei Division from December 2017 to March 2020. She was senior researcher of the Health Promotion Administration, Ministry of Health and Welfare from January 2016 to December 2017. In July 2010, she became the chief of Emergency Care Section, Department of Medical Affairs, Ministry of Health and Welfare. Taipei Division serves more than one-third of the population in Taiwan, ranking its service volume first among the six divisions of the NHIA. The service targets of Taipei Division include nearly 10,000 NHI-contracted hospital and clinics and more than 360,000 insured units. Because of the high density of medical centers in the area, the medical expenses that Taipei Division oversees reached more than NTD 251.1 billion, which accounts for one-third of the amount of Taiwan, and the insurance premium income it collects reaches more than NTD 230 billion. It is particularly worth mentioning that her dedication to work has won her an Exemplary Civil Service Award twice during her career. She is committed to passing on her extensive work experience and knowledge to the younger generation.

Hsueh-Yung (Mary) Tai, M.S. is the director of Medical Review and Pharmaceutical Benefits Division, the NHIA of the Ministry of Health and Welfare, Taiwan. She is a pharmacist, graduating from National Taiwan University with a master's degree in pharmacology. Hsueh-Yung first worked as a medical journalist on *China Times* and then began working in the government. In the 1990s, she was elected to join training programs for the NHI in Canada and the USA. From 1991 to 2017, Hsueh-Yung oversaw the management and regulation of pharmaceuticals, including drug safety assessment, generic products, and regulatory affairs. She got promoted to the deputy director of the Division of Medicinal Products, Taiwan Food and Drug Administration (TFDA) and further served as the director of the Division of Planning and Research Development in the TFDA. Hsueh-Yung joined the NHIA in 2017 and has served as the Director of Medical Review and Pharmaceutical Benefits Division. She was more than glad to return to the field of NHI once again 2 decades after she first got in touch with this field. Dedicating herself to pharmaceutical reimbursement and medical review, she finds it very meaningful to ensure the rational allocation of medical resources and bring the greatest benefits to people in Taiwan.

Yu-Yun Tung, L.L.M. is the deputy director of the Provider Inspection Unit of the NHIA. She holds a master's degree in law from National Taiwan Ocean University and obtained a lawyer's license in 2006. She has 20 years of experience in the field of law and is proficient in the laws and regulations of the NHI. Her main responsibilities in the NHIA are to detect fraudulent medical expenses, resolve violations, and refer persons involved in criminal offense to the court.

Joyce Tsung-Hsi Wang, M.D., M.P.H., Ph.D. holds a medical degree from Taipei Medical University, a master's degree in management of healthcare organization and administration, an Executive MBA, and a PhD degree in occupational medicine and industrial hygiene from National Taiwan University. She is also a gynecologist specializing in healthcare administration and management, healthcare industry development, crisis communication and response, healthcare quality and patient safety, and occupational medicine. Dr. Wang is currently the director of the Planning Division of the NHIA, overseeing the implementation of the virtual NHI card and the health-related aspects of the Smart Government. Prior to that, she was the Director-General of Public Health Bureau in Hsinchu City, Taiwan, and led the planning, coordination, and execution of a wide-range of health policies. She personally engaged in COVID-19 prevention at its onset and the resilient healthcare system constructed by her successfully prevented COVID-19 from spreading in Hsinchu City. From 2018 to 2019, she served as the representative of the Taiwan Ministry of Health and Welfare in Washington D.C. in the United States and successfully facilitated bilateral health and welfare cooperation and communication between high-level officials. The Memorandum of Understanding on health between the two countries was initiated in her tenure. As the first female secretary general of the Ministry of Health and Welfare from 2016 to 2018, she supervised and oversaw important national policies.

Shwu-Huey Wu, M.S. is the director of the Information Management Division of the NHIA, and she oversees the development of the information systems and related IT policies of Taiwan's National Health Insurance system. Director Wu has worked at the NHIA for more than 27 years. She has participated in many NHI programs since its launch date and was in charge of designing the medical claim electronic data file format and maintaining medical payment-related computer software systems from 1995 to 2001. She was also in charge of implementing the first generation of the NHIA's enterprise data warehouse system in 1997. When the NHIA changed the NHI paper card into the NHI IC card, she acted as the main IT contact window of the healthcare smart card project, coordinating IT-related issues from 2002 to 2004. With the development of health insurance policies at various stages and the advancement of information technology, she led the IT team to develop various information systems to improve operational efficiency. During the COVID-19 outbreak in 2020, the TOCC information system was used to help the CECC quickly share the epidemic information with all medical providers. She earned her master's degree at the State University of New York at Binghamton and a bachelor's degree at National Taiwan University.

About the Editors

Po-Chang Lee, M.D., M.T.L. is the director general of the National Health Insurance Administration at the Ministry of Health and Welfare, Taiwan, in Taipei, Taiwan.

Joyce Tsung-Hsi Wang, M.D., M.P.H., Ph.D. is the director of the Planning Division, National Health Insurance Administration, at the Ministry of Health and Welfare, Taiwan, in Taipei, Taiwan.

Tzu-Yu Chen, M.S. is the associate researcher of the Information Management Division, National Health Insurance Administration, at the Ministry of Health and Welfare, Taiwan, in Taipei, Taiwan.

Chia-Hui Peng, M.P.H. is the specialist of the Planning Division, National Health Insurance Administration, at the Ministry of Health and Welfare, Taiwan, in Taipei, Taiwan.

Abbreviations

AI	Artificial intelligence
ALK	Anaplastic lymphoma kinase
ALS	Amyotrophic lateral sclerosis
API	Application Programming Interface
ATM	Automatic teller machine operation
Bipolar TURP	Bipolar transurethral resection
CDC	Centers for Disease Control
CDSS	Clinical decision support system
CECC	Central Epidemic Command Center
CNS	Chinese National Standards
CR	Complete response
CT	Computed tomography
DET	Drug expenditure target
DNR	Do not resuscitate
DRGs	Diagnosis-related groups
EGFR	Epidermal growth factor receptor
GDP	Gross Domestic Product
GDPR	General Data Protection Regulation
HBeAg	Hepatitis B e-antigen
HIPAA	Health Insurance Portability and Accountability Act
HIS	Hospital Information System
HTA	Health Technology Assessment
HTR	Health Technology Reassessment
ICT	Information and communication technology
ICU	Intensive care unit
IDS	Integrated Delivery System
INR	International normalized ratio
ISMS	Information Security Management System
ISO	International Organization for Standardization
MEA	Managed Entry Agreement
MOHW	Ministry of Health and Welfare

MOI	Ministry of the Interior
MRI	Magnetic resonance imaging
NGS	Next-generation sequencing
NHI Express App	National Health Insurance Mobile Easy Access mobile application
NHI MediCloud System	National Health Insurance MediCloud System
NHI	National Health Insurance
NHIA	National Health Insurance Administration
NHIC	National Health Insurance Committee
NHS	National Health System
NIIS	National Immunization Information System
NSAIDs	Nonsteroidal anti-inflammatory drugs
NTD	New Taiwan dollar
NYHA	New York Heart Association
OECD	Organization for Economic Co-operation and Development
PACS	Picture-Archiving and Communication System
PBRS	Pharmaceutical Benefit and Reimbursement Scheme
PDA	Patient decision aids
PDCA	Plan-Do-Check-Act
PDPA	Personal Data Protection Act
PE	Pharmacoeconomics
PR	Partial response
PVA	Price–volume agreement
RVU	Relative value unit
RWD	Real-world data
SCO	Security Operation Center
SD	Stable disease
SDK	Software Development Kit
SMA	Spinal muscular atrophy
TAVI	Transcatheter aortic valve implantation
TFDA	Taiwan Food and Drug Administration
TOCC	Travel history, occupation, contact history, and cluster
TUVP	Transurethral vaporization of the prostate
TVGH	The Taipei Veterans General Hospital
Tw-DRGs	Taiwan diagnosis-related groups
UHC	Universal Health Coverage
VAD	Ventricular assist device
VDI	Virtual Desktop Infrastructure
VPN	Virtual private network
WHO	World Health Organization

Chapter 1
Introduction to the National Health Insurance of Taiwan

Po-Chang Lee

The Core Concepts of Taiwan's National Health Insurance

Taiwan's National Health Insurance (NHI) programme was launched on 1 March 1995 to provide healthcare insurance for all residents. Over 23 million people are living in Taiwan, and over 16% of the population is over the age of 65. The Gross Domestic Product (GDP) per capita of Taiwan exceeded US$ 28,000 in 2020, and the total health expenditure was 6.54% of GDP in 2019. The life expectancy in Taiwan was 84.7 years for women and 78.1 years for men in 2020 (Table 1.1).

Prior to the implementation of the NHI, Taiwan had 13 social insurance schemes, such as labour, government employees' health insurance and farmers insurance, which provided composite social security benefits, including healthcare coverage, to specific groups (Fig. 1.1). However, only 59% of the population was covered by these insurance plans in 1994.

Since the NHI was established, the health component of the aforementioned insurances' healthcare plans was consolidated into the NHI to provide nationwide health protection to Taiwan's citizens and international residents. To improve the quality of health care, ensure the soundness of finance and encourage public participation, 'the second-generation NHI' was launched on 1 January 2013.

P.-C. Lee (✉)
National Health Insurance Administration, Ministry of Health and Welfare, Taiwan, Taipei, Taiwan
e-mail: pochang@nhi.gov.tw

© The Author(s) 2022
P.-C. Lee et al. (eds.), *Digital Health Care in Taiwan*,
https://doi.org/10.1007/978-3-031-05160-9_1

Table 1.1 Profile of Taiwan

Population	23.56 million
Land area	36,197 km²
Ageing (over 65)	16.07%
GDP per capita	US$ 28,180 (nominal)
Crude birth rate Crude death rate	7.01‰ 7.34‰
Infant mortality Maternal mortality	3.6‰ 13.0 0/0000
NHE as % of GDP (2019)	6.54%
Life expectancy	84.7 (F)/78.1(M)

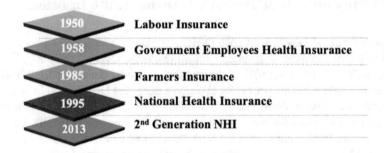

Fig. 1.1 Taiwan's major social insurance programmes

The Organisational Structure and History of the National Health Insurance Administration

The National Health Insurance Administration (NHIA) was previously known as the 'Bureau of National Health Insurance, Department of Health, Executive Yuan'. When the Bureau was merged in 1995, only approximately 59% of the citizens were eligible to participate in the three major occupation-based medical insurance systems—labour insurance, farmers' insurance and government employee health insurance. In line with the principles of financial sustainability and caring for the disadvantaged, these insurance systems were merged and enlarged to become a social insurance system to cover everyone. The Bureau of NHI was repositioned in 2010 as an 'administrative agency' and renamed the NHIA in 2013.

The NHI is a government-run social insurance scheme and is governed by the Ministry of Health and Welfare (MOHW). The MOHW established the NHI Committee to assist with the planning of NHI policies and supervise the implementation of insurance matters. It also established the NHI Mediation Committee to handle disputes concerning health insurance. As the insurer, the NHIA bears responsibility for NHI operations, healthcare quality and information management, research and development as well as personnel training. Administrative funding is provided by the central government through a budgetary process.

To effectively promote various NHI services, in addition to establishing special-ised departments and offices for various services and policy promotions, the NHIA has also established six regional divisions throughout Taiwan, which directly handle underwriting, insurance premium collection, medical expense review and approval as well as the management of contracted medical institutions. Moreover, the NHIA has established 22 contact offices to serve the local residents. As of 30 June 2020, the NHIA had 3125 employees (Fig.1.2).

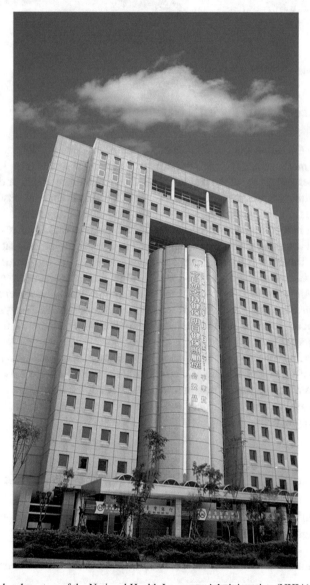

Fig. 1.2 The headquarters of the National Health Insurance Administration (NHIA) in Taipei

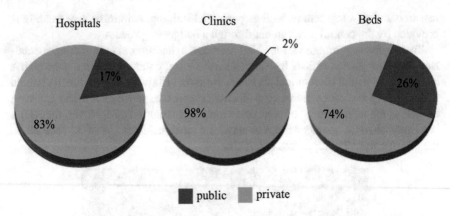

Fig. 1.3 Taiwan's healthcare delivery system

Characteristics of Taiwan's National Health Insurance

Taiwan's healthcare system is dominated by the private sector. Hospitals adopt the closed-staff model, and physicians are primarily paid by hospitals (Fig. 1.3). There is no gatekeeper system to screen patients. Patients can go to any clinic or directly visit a hospital without a referral. Thus, the volume of hospital outpatient services is high. However, health care is usually provided promptly, and waiting time is negligible.

The NHI is a compulsory programme that all citizens and legal residents must join. The NHIA is the only agency authorised to administer the programme, which means that Taiwan's NHI is a single-payer system run by the government. The NHIA collects premiums from the insured, their employers and the government. Premiums comprise 89% of the NHI revenues, out of which the government share is 36% according to the NHI Act. Moreover, the insured make co-payments when using healthcare services and the healthcare providers file claims with the NHIA for reimbursement (Fig. 1.4).

Although it is voluntary for healthcare providers to participate in this programme, about 93% of providers nationwide have joined the NHI. Providers are reimbursed according to plural payment programmes under the global budget payment system. Premium subsidies and co-payment waivers have been granted to the disadvantaged through different projects.

The Finance of the National Health Insurance in Taiwan

As discussed in detail in Chap. 2, the NHI is primarily financed through premiums, including general and supplementary premiums.

Each person remits the general premium according to the premium formula or the fixed figures. The insured are grouped into six categories and are subject to

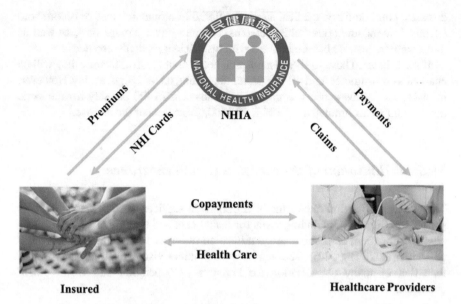

Fig. 1.4 The framework of the National Health Insurance

different premium calculation bases and contribution shares, depending on the category that they belong to. Most salaried employees have to pay 30% of their premiums, with their employers paying 60% and the government paying the remaining 10%. The government subsidises 100% of the premiums for low-income households and military conscripts. Inmates are also covered under the NHI, and their premiums are paid by the government.

In the first decade of the twenty-first century, salary income as a percentage of national income declined, making premium growth lag behind income growth, thereby leading to funding shortfalls. The introduction of the supplementary premium on various types of incomes, other than regular payroll, has alleviated the perennial financial problems. Since 2013, in addition to the general premium, a supplementary premium has also been collected. The insured are charged a supplementary premium of 2.11% on certain incomes they receive, including large bonuses, professional fees, part-time wages, stock dividends, interest income and rental income.

The NHI provides comprehensive benefits that cover inpatient care, outpatient care, drugs, dental services, traditional Chinese medicine, day care for the mentally ill and home-based medical care. Moreover, expensive health services, such as dialysis and organ transplants, are all covered.

The insured make co-payments for their outpatient care to avoid the unnecessary utilisation of medical resources. The co-payment is partially waived if the outpatient visit is arranged by a referral. To ensure that people who need health care are not denied access because of the cost-sharing mechanism, individuals who meet certain conditions are exempt from co-payments, such as patients with catastrophic diseases, child delivery, medical services offered in mountain areas or on offshore islands, low-income households, veterans, children under the age of 3, as well as those who are insured but are in areas with insufficient medical resources.

If those insured have to stay in a hospital because of medical factors, they will be charged a co-insurance, and the rate varies depending on the length of stay. However, in 2021, this co-insurance was capped at around US$ 1400 per stay for the same disease and an accumulated total of US$ 2400, regardless of the disease.

Medical Utilisation of the National Health Insurance

The average utilisation rate of the NHI outpatient services in 2020 was 14.2 visits per person (Fig. 1.5), including visits for dental care and traditional Chinese medicine. For inpatient care, the average utilisation rate was 14.12 admissions per 100 persons in 2020 (Fig. 1.6). The number of outpatient visits is substantially higher than that of many Organisation for Economic Cooperation and Development countries.

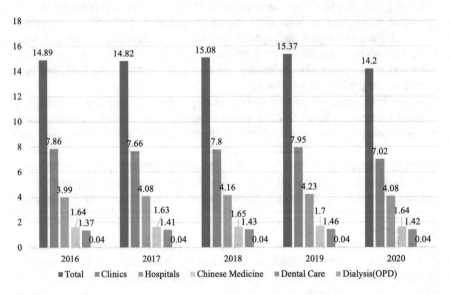

Fig. 1.5 Outpatient visits per person

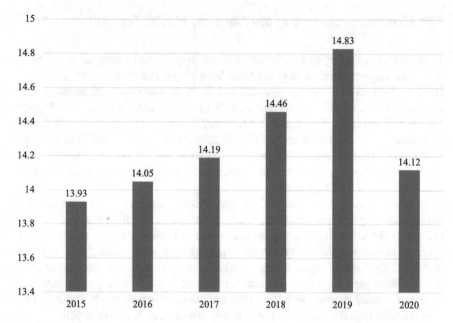

Fig. 1.6 Number of hospital admissions per 100 persons

The Payment System of the National Health Insurance

When the NHI system was initiated, it sought to quickly integrate the existing civil service, labour and farmers' insurance systems. The fee-for-service approach was adopted as the primary payment system. Moreover, using the government and labour insurance payment standards as the basis, the NHI's payment standards were revised, and the scope of reimbursements and recommendations of medical groups were adjusted. However, this system resulted in an uncontrolled increase in medical expenses and has affected the quality of care. The NHIA has followed the example of other leading countries by designing different payment methods based on the characteristics of different types of medical care. The NHIA built the global budget payment systems, including global budgets for dental care, Chinese medicine, clinics, hospitals and dialysis. To further rationalise the reimbursement of health services, a resource-based relative value scale and a Taiwanese version of diagnosis-related groups (DRGs) were initiated in 2004 and 2010 respectively. The payment system of the NHI is discussed in more detail in Chap. 3.

The Healthcare Quality of the National Health Insurance

To enhance the quality of health care, various projects addressing different needs have been implemented to offer adequate health care. For example, the Integrated Delivery System Plan, which was initiated in 1999, has improved health care in mountainous areas and on offshore islands by encouraging hospitals to dispatch doctors to these areas. This Integrated Delivery System Plan provides health care to 50 remote areas and serves about 480,000 people each year. In addition, different pay-for-performance projects have been implemented for certain diseases since 2001. Furthermore, patient-centred projects are effective to make patients easily access the health care they need.

For those who are less fortunate, the government provides several types of assistance, such as premium subsidies, financial assistance for the poor and medical assistance for the disadvantaged, to make sure that they have access to medical services. In addition, the policy of unlocking NHI cards removes the fetters imposed on financially disadvantaged people who fear seeking medical care because of overdue premium payments. One of the core values of Taiwan's NHI programme is to remove financial barriers in health care for people through the NHI fund. This explains why the NHI can cover catastrophic diseases, such as haemophilia, which makes a patient cost 97 times as much as the average patient. The strategies for pursuing health equity through the NHI will be introduced in Chap. 5.

The Information System of the National Health Insurance

The NHI MediCloud system provides medical professionals with patients' medical data to ensure drug safety and enhance healthcare quality. Medical professionals use the system online to view patients' previous important data and images when patients visit them or are hospitalised. Medical professionals can read patients' records of medications, surgeries, tests and exams, medical images, history of drug allergies, etc., through a secure virtual private network.

Figure 1.7 depicts the reduction rates of overlapping medication with the use of the NHI MediCloud system. In terms of overlapping days, the prescriptions of six selected drugs for chronic diseases with the same pharmacological action have significantly decreased by over half from 2014 to 2020, resulting in not only a savings of more than US$ 10 million but also making patients safer.

Furthermore, the NHI MediCloud system can improve the utilisation efficiency of medical resources. Physicians can view patients' medical images, such as computed tomography (CT) scans, magnetic resonance imaging (MRI), X-rays, ultrasound images and endoscopic images, uploaded by other healthcare providers.

Smart card technology has been adopted since 1 January 2004. The NHI card contains records of a patient's last six visits, drug prescriptions, drug allergies, catastrophic diseases, consent for organ donation, consent to palliative care and consent

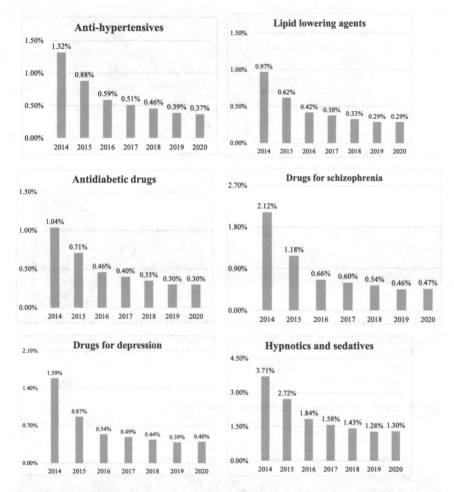

Fig. 1.7 The overlapping rates of medication with the use of the National Health Insurance MediCloud system

to a 'Do not resuscitate' (DNR) order (Fig. 1.8). The NHI card can also be used to monitor high-utilisation patients and detect fraud by analysing data that are uploaded daily. It can also help to identify potential carriers of communicable diseases in major epidemic outbreaks. Over the years, cloud computing technology has also been applied to give the card additional and more powerful functions, and the Virtual NHI Card Pilot Plan is also underway (Fig. 1.9).

To heighten awareness of self-care and preventive health care, 'My Health Bank' was established. People can initiate their 'My Health Bank' account by authenticating themselves on a mobile phone or computer to access their health data anytime anywhere. 'My Health Bank' provides people with 3 years of medical data, medication records, test and exam results, vaccination records, as well as other useful services, including online named-based medical mask purchases (Fig. 1.10).

- Last Six Medical Visits
- Drug Prescriptions and
  Allergies
- Catastrophic Diseases
- Organ Donation Consent
- Palliative Care
- DNR

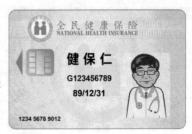

Fig. 1.8 The records on the National Health Insurance card

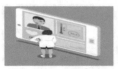 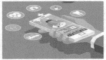 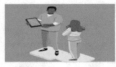 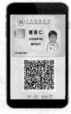

NHI Administration	**Insured**	**Healthcare Providers**	**Virtual NHI Card**

• Data management
• Infectious disease
  tracing &
  monitoring
	• Identification
	• Paper cards
	  consolidated
		• Authentication	• One-time only
			  QR-CODE
			• Pilot Plan
			  underway

Fig. 1.9 The Virtual National Health Insurance Card Pilot Plan

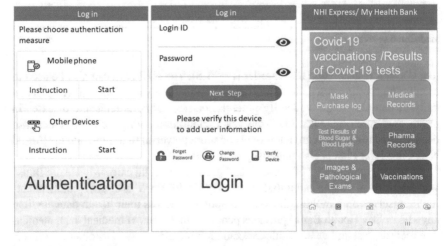

Fig. 1.10 My Health Bank

Table 1.2 Digital technologies in response to COVID-19

Big data	MediCloud	National Health Insurance card
Analyse medical data for pandemic surveillance	A real-time alert for healthcare professionals when providing health care	For name-based medical mask purchase For vaccination registrations and reservations

To prevent COVID-19 from spreading to communities during its early phase, since January 2020, the NHI MediCloud system has served as a real-time alert for healthcare providers. For any person with defined conditions, including foreign travel history, designated occupation, contact with a COVID-19 patient and a specific clustering situation, the NHI MediCloud system allows healthcare providers to obtain these data in real time and pay the costs for health care, enabling efficient triage as well as rapid and accurate diagnoses.

Moreover, the NHI card is used for name-based medical mask purchase. People can go to pharmacies to buy government-supplied medical masks with their NHI cards. This system helped people to have access to medical masks at the beginning of the pandemic when there was a shortage of medical masks. The NHIA also releases data on mask sales timely to cooperate with non-profit groups to update their 'mask purchase map' apps. The NHIA also analyses and provides medical data to Taiwan's Centers for Disease Control, MOHW for pandemic surveillance (Table 1.2).

The NHIA has a huge health database with a grand collection of medical images and data. To facilitate the development of artificial intelligence (AI) models for health care, researchers can apply to use these de-identified CT and MRI images to develop AI for precision medicine applications to enhance the quality of health care. Several successful applications have been developed, including MedChex, a detection platform for COVID-19 with an accuracy rate of 92%; DeepMets+, a diagnostic model with an accuracy rate of 97% in detecting brain tumours and metastatic lesions; PANCREASaver, which automatically identifies pancreatic cancer with an accuracy rate of up to 91.1%. Moreover, the NHIA uses a cloud-computing platform for data cleaning, image labelling and data training to build a basis of value-added NHI big data and facilitate analysis and research.

Achievement of the National Health Insurance

The NHI has earned a good reputation among citizens of Taiwan and is considered to be one of Taiwan's most popular public programmes. The public satisfaction rate has improved from 39% in 1995, the NHI programme's first year, to 61% in its second year and to more than 80% recently. According to a poll in 2020, public satisfaction with the NHI programme is 90.2% (Fig. 1.11).

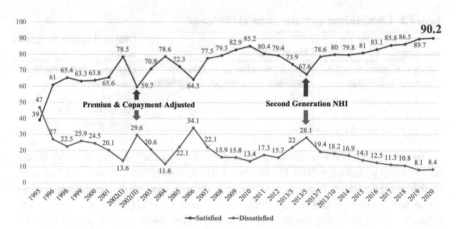

Fig. 1.11 The high public satisfaction with the National Health Insurance programme

The NHI has safeguarded the health of all nationals and residents since its inception. People are insured to have easy access to healthcare providers regardless of their ability to pay. The NHI has not only established a secure healthcare network for all residents in Taiwan but is also well-known internationally for achieving universal health coverage and providing comprehensive health care at an affordable cost. Public satisfaction is also high, and medical quality is assured.

The NHI plays a crucial role in improving people's health in Taiwan and has been sharing its successful experience with the rest of the world. However, the challenges it faces include rising life expectancies, increased prevalence of chronic diseases, technological advancement, as well as new drugs, which stimulate more innovative solutions. Therefore, 'My Health Bank' and the NHI MediCloud system were established to ensure the quality of health care and strengthen people's health. Furthermore, virtual NHI card and AI technology are currently applied to some pilot projects to achieve high-performing, efficient and secure operations.

The Critical Blueprints of Taiwan's National Health Insurance

The outbreak of coronavirus disease has created a global health crisis that has had a deep impact on the way we perceive our world and everyday lives. Some countries were caught off guard by the sudden epidemic and struggled with disaster reduction. Taiwan employed the "National Health Insurance MediCloud System (NHI MediCloud System)" immediately as a platform to instantly update patient travel histories. This initial prevention measure received a positive response from the medical field. *BMJ Opinion*, the top international academic journal, published an article on 21 July 2020, titled "What we can learn from Taiwan's response to the COVID-19 epidemic?". It explained Taiwan's use of medical information technology and

Apply AI to NHI Big Data

- All the data was de-identified to protect personal privacy for application
- Development of precision medicine and precise claim review

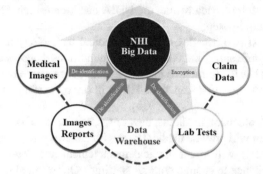

Fig. 1.12 Applying artificial intelligence to National Health Insurance big data

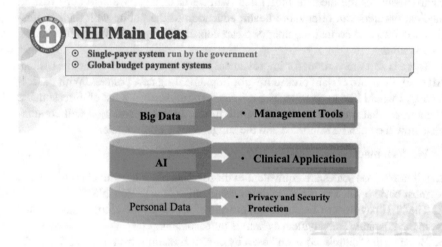

Fig. 1.13 Main ideas of National Health Insurance

comprehensive medical information to facilitate a farsighted project to face the contagious disease.

With the breakthroughs and continuous development of science and technology each year, an artificial intelligence (AI) wave has been sweeping the globe. Taiwan's National Health Insurance (NHI) system has accumulated a medical claims database for 27 years, which is the best foundation for developing AI applications and big data analyses for health care (Figs. 1.12 and 1.13) to gradually develop new medical economic models.

Taiwan has a strong and solid information technology background that can create a smart telemedicine model through information and communication network technology so that medical care is no longer limited by distance. In addition, "home-based medical care" is a new trend. Taiwan's National Health Insurance Administration (NHIA) encourages medical personnel to join the medical team. It is believed that more new medical technologies will be applied to home-based medical care in the future. Meanwhile, the NHIA has been establishing a new management system step by step.

Over the past two decades, although medical technology and equipment have progressed significantly, patients' clinical conditions have become increasingly complex. This has led to relative increases in labour resource requirements in practising treatments. As a first step, the NHIA will review system fairness and payment standards.

Medical AI, precision medicine, new drugs, new medical devices and new medical technologies will provide medical care with a new economic model. These medical developments will affect medical management and new business strategies. "There is no chance to change without starting". Our original goal at the outset, to provide the best medical care for 23 million people and create a happy working environment for the medical profession, will never change. We also hope that all medical partners can offer more health education to the public with their professional knowledge so that together, we can conserve the precious resources of the NHI system.

There is still much room for improvement in our system, but it cannot be rushed. After all, there are certain procedures for implementing new policies. With the following, I would like to provide, as a reference for all sectors, a list of unreasonable phenomena that must be dealt with in the future. In the meantime, I will contemplate how they can be improved and the suggestions I would make.

Western medicine clinics

1. Clinics whose scales are equivalent to those of hospitals are still classified at the most basic level. The global budget classification is unreasonable.
2. The NHI payment of the "medical examination fee" in the clinic is higher than in the hospital. The payment system is unreasonable.
3. Because the "simplified form" used by clinics is exempt from review, the medication prescription information uploaded by clinics is incomplete.

Hospital

1. The annual growth in some "specialties" exceeds the Negotiated Global Budget Growth Rate for the year, thus squeezing low-growth specialties.
2. The new hospital establishment approved by the Ministry of Health and Welfare induces demand for medical treatment and affects NHI finances.
3. The biggest beneficiary of the National Health Insurance payment system is the hospital operator. And the medical personnel who actually provide the service have not been treated reasonably.
4. The hospital was punished for doctors' violations of the regulations. The scope of the collective punishment currently includes statutory specialties and should be reviewed.

Institutional elements

1. Medical affairs

    (a) Under the same global budget category, relative value units (RVUs) are different under the jurisdiction of each regional division of the NHIA.
    (b) Institutions in "regions in remote areas with insufficient medical resources" should be recognised based on facts.
    (c) The newly obtained "nursing fee", "transplant coordinator fee" and others were not actually paid to the service providers.
    (d) Does the calculation formula for the annual growth of the global budget of NHI meet the actual conditions?
    (e) The requirements for NHI-contracted medical institutions are loose. The excessive supply of hospitals and clinics indirectly induces medical demand.
    (f) Has the "overseas medical reimbursement system" become a loophole?

2. Medical review and investigation

    (a) How to stop investigating cases that have already occurred and avoid recurrences?
    (b) Is the intricate relationship between hospitals and "long-term care facilities" a major loophole?

3. Drug payment

    (a) Have the drugs for rare diseases been controlled by specific hospitals and doctors?
    (b) There are too many drug items in the NHI system, and an exit mechanism or a competition mechanism should be established.

Chapter 2
Income Strategy

Po-Chang Lee, Mei-Hsin Chen, Shu-Ching Chiang, and Yu-Pin Chang

Introduction

National Health Insurance (NHI) is compulsory social insurance that adopts an independent financial system. The government bears the statutory obligation for the premiums but is not responsible for filling the income gap. Therefore, a stable and sufficient source of insurance income is the cornerstone of the sustainable operation of NHI.

Sources of National Health Insurance Income

During the early stage of the NHI, premiums were calculated and collected based on regular salary income. As salaries have grown at a slower rate than medical expenditures, the financial gap of NHI has gradually expanded. To improve the financial condition and increase the fairness of premium contributions, besides actively seeking supplementary financial resources, the National Health Insurance Administration (NHIA) implemented the second generation of NHI in 2013. It began collecting "supplementary premiums" for non-recurring salary income and increased the government's overall contribution rate. Therefore, NHI income currently comes from premiums as well as other insurance income.

P.-C. Lee (✉) · M.-H. Chen · S.-C. Chiang · Y.-P. Chang
National Health Insurance Administration, Ministry of Health and Welfare, Taiwan, Taipei, Taiwan
e-mail: pochang@nhi.gov.tw; meihsin@nhi.gov.tw; grace7@nhi.gov.tw; A110413@nhi.gov.tw

© The Author(s) 2022 17
P.-C. Lee et al. (eds.), *Digital Health Care in Taiwan*,
https://doi.org/10.1007/978-3-031-05160-9_2

Premium Income

National Health Insurance premium income includes regular premiums, supplementary premiums, and a 36% difference contributed by the government. Regular
premiums are billed according to the occupation and salary of the insured. For
instance, the insured classified within categories 1, 2 and 3 are employees, and their
premiums are calculated based on their monthly salaries. The insured classified
within categories 4, 5 and 6 pay premiums calculated based on the average premiums of the insured in categories 1–3, and a fixed insurance premium is charged. The
calculation of supplementary premiums includes large bonuses, part-time wages,
professional service income, dividend income, interest income, rental income and
the difference between the total monthly salaries paid by employers (the insured
units) and the total payroll basis of the employees. In addition, the current premiums
are paid by the insured, the insured units, and the government at the statutory rate,
and the NHI Act specifies that the government's contribution to annual premiums
must be at least 36% of the total. Therefore, when the government's contribution is
less than 36%, other budgets must be allocated to make up for it. Other insurance
income includes tobacco health and welfare surcharges, public welfare lottery earnings that are distributed to reserve funds by law, overdue charges for late payments
of premiums and net investment income.

Proportions of Various Sources of Income

The analysis is based on the NHI system's income sources in 2020 (Fig. 2.1). Total
insurance income is New Taiwan dollars (NTD) 627.8 billion. The premium income
(comprising regular premiums, supplementary premiums and the 36% difference
contributed by the government) is NTD 614.3 billion, accounting for 98% of total
revenue, and it is the main source of income. Other income is NTD 13.5 billion,

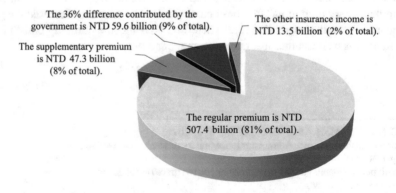

Fig. 2.1 The amounts and proportions of various sources of insurance income in 2020

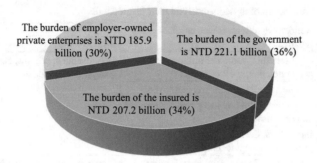

Fig. 2.2 The amount and proportion of the tripartite burden of premium income in 2020

accounting for only 2% of total revenue. The tripartite premium burdens of the insured, employer-owned private enterprises and the government (Fig. 2.2) accounted for NTD 207.2 billion (34%), NTD 185.9 billion (30%) and NTD 221.1 billion (36%).

Enrolment Eligibility and Premium Calculations

The NHI provides universal coverage to all citizens of Taiwan who have previously participated in the NHI within the last 2 years and have a registered domicile in the Taiwan area. Those who have had a registered domicile in the Taiwan area for 6 months, and any person with an alien resident certificate for the Taiwan area who has resided in Taiwan for at least 6 months must participate in the NHI and pay premiums, whether staying in Taiwan or abroad. The right of the insured to access medical care is protected, whether they suffer from illness or injury or require reproductive care. Since the implementation of Taiwan's NHI, it has undergone several revisions to gradually expand its coverage to nationals with a registered domicile, new immigrants, foreigners stationed long term in Taiwan, overseas Chinese and foreign students, military personnel, and inmates at correctional facilities.

Classification of the Insured

The NHI classifies insureds into six categories based on occupation, status and some specific groups to which they may belong. Categories 1–4 classify those insured by their occupational groups; category 5 consists of members of low-income households; and category 6 consists of veterans or dependents of deceased veterans and heads of households or household representatives other than the abovementioned insured and their dependents. The insured should participate in the NHI system in order of eligibility from category 1 to category 6 (Table 2.1).

Table 2.1 Classification of those insured and their insured units

Category	National Health Insurance enrolees (insured)	Insured units
Category 1	Civil servants, volunteer military personnel, public office holders	Organisations, schools, companies, groups, or individuals
	Private school teachers and employees	
	Employees of public and private enterprises and organisations	
	Employers, the self-employed, independent professionals and technical specialists	
Category 2	Occupational union members, foreign crew members	Occupational unions, the Master Mariners Associations, the National Chinese Seamen's unions
Category 3	Members of farmers' and fishermen's associations actually engaged in agricultural and fishery work	Farmers' associations, fishermen's associations
Category 4	Conscripted servicemen, students in military schools, dependents of military service members on pensions	Agencies designated by the Ministry of National Defence
	Males performing alternative military service	Agencies designated by the Ministry of the Interior
	Inmates at correctional facilities	Agencies designated by the Ministry of Justice
Category 5	Members of low-income households as defined by the Public Assistance Act	Administrative office of the household is registered
Category 6	Veterans or dependents of deceased veterans	Administrative office of the household is registered
	Heads of households or household representatives	

Calculation of Premiums

The NHI premiums adopt the principle of ability to pay, and the computation varies according to the category of those insured. The premium paid by the insured (the public), the insured units (employers), and the government is divided into regular premiums and supplementary premiums (Table 2.2).

1. Premiums of those insured:

   (a) Regular premium. The regular premium is calculated based on income from labour services such as regular wages; the dependents' premiums are paid by those insured, and the maximum number of dependents is three, even if the actual number is higher.

   (b) Supplementary premium. The second generation of NHI was implemented on 1 January 2013. Items such as large bonuses, part-time wages, professional service income, dividend income, interest income and rental income not included in calculating the regular premium are included in the billing

Table 2.2 Calculation of National Health Insurance premiums

Premium of insured = regular premium + supplementary premium	
Regular premium	Categories 1–3: salary basis × regular premium rate × contribution ratio × (1 + number of dependents) The maximum number of dependents is three, even if the actual number is higher. Categories 4–6: fixed premium
Supplementary premium	Supplementary premium is collected from Categories 1–4 and Category 6: (high bonuses, part-time wages, professional service income, stock dividends, interest income, rental income) × supplementary premium rate Notes: Category 5 low-income households are exempt from contributing supplementary premiums
Premium of insured unit = regular premium + supplementary premium	
Regular premium	Category 1, items 1–3: salary basis × regular premium rate × contribution ratio × (1 + average number of dependents)
Supplementary premium	The supplementary premium is collected from Category 1, items 1–3: (total monthly salaries that employers actually pay their employees – total salary basis of employees) × supplementary premium rate

Notes:
1. Effective January 2021, the regular premium rate is 5.17%, and the supplementary premium rate is 2.11%.
2. Part-time wages—wage income not paid by the insurance registration organisation of those insured.

> basis for supplementary premium. Expanding the premium base can ensure that persons with equivalent incomes pay similar premiums, thus improving the fairness of the burden.

2. Premiums of insured units

    (a) Regular premium. The regular premium is calculated based on labour income such as regular employee wages.

    (b) Supplementary premium. The supplementary premium is collected on the difference between the total monthly salaries that employers actually pay their employees each month and the total payroll basis for those employees.

Calculation of the Premium Rate

To maintain the financial independence and liability system of the NHI, the National Health Insurance Act stipulates that the annual premium rate should be reviewed each year. In principle, the total amount of the NHI reserve fund must be at least 1–3 months of insurance payments. Hence, the actuarial calculation plays a crucial role in reviewing the annual premium rate.

The Annual Premium Rate Review Process

Following the second generation of NHI implementation, the annual premium rate review process has gradually applied an income/expenditure linkage mechanism. The National Health Insurance Committee (NHIC), comprising the insured, employers, insurance medical service providers, experts, reputable public figures, and representatives from relevant agencies, negotiates the total amount of the next year's global budget each September. After accounting for the estimated insurance income, the committee decides the annual premium rate. Because the annual premium rate has to be announced within certain time frame, the National Health Insurance Act stipulates that the NHIC must complete the rate review process 1 month before the start of the next year and submit it to the Ministry of Health and Welfare (MOHW) to obtain the Executive Yuan's approval. If the annual premium rate review process cannot be completed within the specified time, the MOHW will submit the suggested rate for the Executive Yuan's approval (Fig. 2.3):

The Financial Structure of National Health Insurance

The financial structure of NHI is mainly composed of three parts, including the insurance income, the insurance costs and the reserve fund.

Insurance income includes the premium income and other insurance income, which is mainly used to cover the insurance costs such as medical expenses for the insured. Among them, the premiums account for about 98% of the insurance income, which is the most important source for the income of NHI. The premiums include the regular premiums, the supplementary premiums and the 36% difference contributed by the government. Other insurance income includes tobacco health and welfare surcharges, public welfare lottery earnings distributions, overdue charges for the premiums and net investment income.

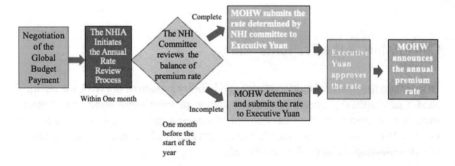

Fig. 2.3 National Health Insurance annual premium rate review procedures

As for the insurance costs, it includes the insurance payment and other insurance costs. Among them, insurance payment accounted for about 99.95% of the insurance costs. It is the total amount of medical benefit payments determined in the agreement, after deducting the expenses borne by the insured, the amount of subrogation compensation and tobacco health and welfare surcharge subsidies for rare-disease medications (Fig. 2.4). Other insurance costs include expenditures for improving the effectiveness of insurance services, small shortfall payment of the premiums and reissuance checks that have not been cashed for more than 2 years.

The function of the reserve fund is to adjust the income and costs of NHI. If there is a balance between the income and costs of the insurance in the current year, the balance shall be deposited into the reserve fund. On the contrary, the reserve fund will be used to fill shortfalls between income and costs (Fig. 2.5).

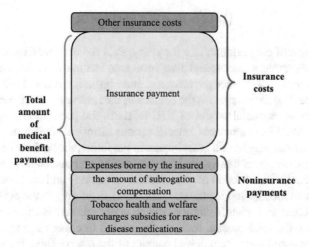

Fig. 2.4 Insurance cost architecture

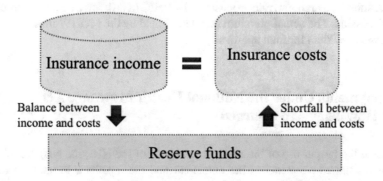

Fig. 2.5 Correlation of the reserve fund, insurance income and insurance costs

Establishment of an Actuarial Model to Calculate the Premium Rate

The NHIA uses three major components of financing NHI to establish the current actuarial model for the premium rate. In accordance with the regulations of the NHI Act, the actuarial calculation of the premium rate adopts the method of "adjust income to expense", and the premium rate is calculated based on the principle of covering insurance costs and maintaining the total reserve fund for 1–3 months of the insurance payment. The description of the model is as follows:

$$Pt(r) = Bt + \Delta St$$

$$St = \Delta St + St - 1$$

$$(1/12) \times Bt < St < (3/12) \times Bt$$

r is the balance of the premium rate for year t. Pt is the insurance income of year t, including the premium income and other insurance income. Bt is the insurance costs for year t, including insurance payment and other insurance costs. ΔSt is the amount of the reserve fund for year t. St is the balance of the reserve fund at the end of year t.

The premium actuarial model of NHI refers to the population projection data from the National Development Council, various historical changes and trends, the major policies that may have a great impact in the future, medical service costs (e.g. new drugs and treatment items), goals of medical policy, reasonable growth of medical expenses, the introduction of new medical technology and other factors to estimate insurance income and insurance costs. Then, according to the pre-set rate, the premium income and other insurance income under this rate is calculated to determine whether the total income this year is enough to cover the annual estimated insurance costs and meet the required amount of the reserve fund. By adjusting the rate value repeatedly in this way to derive the minimum rate value that equates both sides, the balance rate that meets the legal standard for that year is finalised.

According to the trial calculation results of the premium rate actuarial model, the NHIA submits a premium rate proposal to the NHIC (a task force under the MOHW) for discussion. The actual premium rate determined by the MOHW must be sent to the Executive Yuan for final approval.

Co-payments Under the National Health Insurance Act and How They Are Charged

To make the proper use of the medical resources of the NHI, the NHI Act clearly stipulates the co-payments of the outpatient and the inpatient. In addition to the premiums, those insured also need to pay a part of the medical expenses when seeking medical care. This increases the cost awareness of the insured and prevents the insured from using medical resources at will because of paying the premiums. It further reduces unnecessary medical care and enhances the efficiency of the payments.

According to the NHI Act, the outpatient co-payment can be calculated and divided into two systems called the "fixed-rate system" and the "fixed-quota system", and each system has its own advantages and disadvantages. The current outpatient co-payment employs the "fixed-quota system". When NHI was launched 27 years ago, a "fixed-rate system" was considered to pose too-large an economic burden, which would create an economic barrier for economically disadvantaged people seeking medical care. Therefore, in accordance with Article 43, Item 3 of the NHI Act and Article 61 of the Enforcement Rules of the NHI Act, a fixed-quota system was adopted and promulgated to charge a certain amount for the basic outpatient and emergency care co-payments, outpatient medicine co-payments and co-payments for outpatient rehabilitation (including Chinese medicine traumatology) for patients receiving follow-up treatment (apart from the moderate to complex and complex items of the rehabilitation physical therapy), and they have been used until now.

According to the NHI Act, the inpatient co-payment adopts a "fixed-rate system" and charges 5–30% of the inpatient medical expenses depending on the acute and chronic wards and the length of hospitalisation.

Co-payments for Outpatient Visits

At the initial establishment of the NHI, the public did not understand the level of medical institutions and the related operations with or without a referral. Therefore, there was a period when the Western medicine outpatient co-payment could not be determined with or without a referral. On 15 July 2005, the Western medicine outpatient co-payment was set. It is charged according to the level of the medical institution, and there are distinctions between visits with and without referrals.

To promote a tiered medical care system and increase primary medical service capacity, diversions and referrals of patients are based on professional medical opinions to ensure that medical institutions at all levels can perform their duties through the division of work and cooperation in care. The co-payment adjustment plan for the National Health Insurance's outpatient and emergency care was implemented on 15 April 2017. The outpatient co-payment for patients referred to medical centres and regional hospitals has been reduced. However, the outpatient co-payment increases if one goes to a medical centre or regional hospital without a referral. Thus, the current outpatient co-payment structure of the NHI is as follows:

1. Basic co-payment for outpatient visits (Table 2.3): Western medicine outpatients at all levels with and without referral, NTD 170 and NTD 420 for medical centres, NTD 100 and NTD 240 for regional hospitals, NTD 50 and NTD 80 for district hospitals, and NTD 50 for clinics, dental medicine care and Chinese medicine.

Table 2.3 National Health Insurance co-payments for outpatient visits

Type of institution	Western medicine outpatient care		Dental care (NTD)	Chinese medicine (NTD)
	With referral (NTD)	Without referral (NTD)		
Medical centres	170	420	50	50
Regional hospitals	100	240	50	50
District hospitals	50	80	50	50
Clinics	50	50	50	50

Table 2.4 Co-payments for medicines

Prescription costs (NTD)	Co-payments for medicines (NTD)
Under 100	0
101–200	20
201–300	40
301–400	60
401–500	80
501–600	100
601–700	120
701–800	140
801–900	160
901–1000	180
1001 or more	200

2. Co-payment for medicines (Table 2.4): the co-payment is waived for prescription costs less than NTD 100, NTD 20 for each additional NTD 100 of the prescription costs will be charged and the ceiling price is NTD 200. Continuous prescriptions for chronic diseases (prescribed for more than 28 days), dental medical care and case payment items are exempt from medicine co-payments.
3. Outpatient rehabilitation co-payment (including Chinese medicine traumatology) of NTD 50 is charged each time for the same course of treatment from the second time (apart from moderate to complex and complex items of rehabilitation physical therapy).

Co-payments for Emergency Care

In the initial stage of establishing the NHI, the basic co-payment quota for emergency care is set according to the types of medical institutions. The purpose is to make effective use of emergency medical resources in hospitals. In order to return the medical centre to the role of emergency intensive care, the co-payment of emergency care was adjusted on 15 April 2017. To the medical centre's emergency

Table 2.5 Co-payments for emergency care

Type of institution	Emergency care	
	Triage classification	
	Grades 1 & 2 (NTD)	Grades 3, 4 & 5 (NTD)
Medical centres	450	550
Regional hospitals	300	
District hospitals	150	
Clinics	150	

Table 2.6 Co-payment rates for inpatient care

Ward	Co-payment rates			
	5%	10%	20%	30%
Acute	–	30 days or less	31–60 days	61 days or more
Chronic	30 days or less	31–90 days	91–180 days	181 days or more

Table 2.7 Co-payment ceiling per hospitalisation and for the entire year

Year	Co-payment ceiling per hospitalisation (NTD)	Co-payment ceiling for the whole year (NTD)
2021	41,000	69,000
2020	39,000	65,000
2019	39,000	65,000
2018	38,000	64,000
2017	37,000	62,000

department, the co-payment of Grades 3, 4 and 5 of the triage grades are NTD 550, and Grades 1 and 2 are NTD 450 respectively. The co-payment of the regional and district hospitals' emergency care remains at NTD 300 and NTD 150 respectively (Table 2.5), guiding people to change their medical habits and to cherish emergency medical resources.

Co-payment Rates for Inpatient Care

In accordance with Article 47 of the NHI Act, the inpatient co-payment will charge 5–30% of hospitalisation medical expenses according to the acute and chronic wards and the length of hospitalisation (Table 2.6).

The maximum amount of the co-payments to be borne by the insured per hospitalisation in an acute care ward for not more than 30 days or in a chronic ward for not more than 180 days for the same illness and the maximum amount for the accumulated co-payments for the whole year shall be determined by the competent authority (Table 2.7).

The co-payment mechanism in the NHI Act reflects the spirit of social insurance. In every country that implements social insurance, a co-payment system will be formulated to remind everyone that medical resources are precious. Because the medical resource should be used to help people who are sick, it should be spent where it is most needed, and it must be used appropriately.

There are many opinions from all stakeholders regarding the adoption of a "fixed-rate system" or a "fixed-quota system" for co-payment. There is no perfect policy. We can only seek a balance between the tendencies of the policy goals to achieve sub-optimal effects. It is also hoped that the public will realise that "the National Health Insurance is the property of the whole people" and cherish the resources of the NHI.

Fair Burden—Change Unnecessary Health Care [1]

To maintain financial balance and protect disadvantaged groups, the Minister of Health and Welfare, Shih-Chung Chen, increased the premium rate of the NHI from 4.69% to 5.17% in 2021. Then, the annual premium contributed by 890,000 business owners increased by NTD 19.3 billion, and the government's annual expenditure has increased by NTD 23 billion. For about 1.26 million people who originally received full government subsidies, their premiums are still borne by the government. However, such a premium income is still not enough to balance the continuously growing medical expenses. There must be financial management supporting measures to make good use of the resources of the NHI to which everyone contributed.

The Value of National Health Insurance Manifests When Major Illnesses Occur

The financial mechanism of the NHI is that an annual medical global budget is set first, and medical services are paid in relative value units (RVUs). If medical institutions only focus on increasing the number of medical services delivered or drugs prescribed, then the more RVUs exceed the global budget, and the lower the value of the RVUs will be. Moreover, the same medical behaviour will result in a reduced monetary return. Medical ethics is the cornerstone of medical behaviour. We hope to communicate and work with the medical profession and the public, to confront human nature practically, and that the medical profession may contribute high-quality medical services with pleasure.

Academia and medical profession have different opinions on whether Taiwan's NHI is social welfare or social insurance. Some people think that the monthly premiums or supplementary premiums are expensive when they are not in need of medical treatment. However, they realise the core value of the NHI when they or their loved ones have major illnesses.

Provide the Best Drugs for Patients in Need

From 2018 to 2020, the NHIA included 55 new antineoplastic drugs covering 16 types of cancers with the assistance of medical experts. This annual drug expenditure amounts to NTD 12.8 billion. The coverage expansion is estimated to benefit more than 8000 patients each year. At the same time, 20 drugs for rare diseases were also included, with an annual drug expenditure of NTD 1.6 billion, to benefit more than 1000 patients. There is an annual drug expenditure of NTD 3.5 billion for hepatitis B, benefiting about 90,000 patients each year. The accumulated expenditure on new oral drugs for hepatitis C is about NTD 20.2 billion. More than 110,000 patients benefited from the policy.

Only patients will not forget about the physical and mental suffering caused by diseases and the financial pressure caused by striving to obtain the best medical treatment that they and their families can bear. Providing patients who are really in need with the best medication is the priority and goal of the NHIA.

Avoid the Vicious Circle

By analysing outpatient medical expenses, we found that medical personnel's labour income "Diagnostic Fee" only accounts for 17.7%, and the proportion is declining year by year. The "Medication Fee" accounts for 27.2% and the "Examination and Test" accounts for 12.5%, and both proportions are increasing every year. Obviously, many resources are shared by machines and medicines rather than labour and expertise. This ecology is a vicious circle that the NHIA and the medical profession must face seriously.

Therefore, Minister Shih-Chung Chen proposed three major reform directions:

1. Reducing unnecessary medical services. Apply the National Health Insurance MediCloud System (NHI MediCloud System) to promote medical resource sharing and to suppress improper use of medical resources.
2. Fair burden. Review the co-payment system of health care and review the rights and obligations of citizens living abroad.
3. Quality improvement. Integrate the public health system to cover prevention, medical treatment, and the hospice-based palliative care at the end of life.

The essence of the "User Charge" is the "Fair Burden", which is more in line with the concept of health insurance for the young generation who truly bears the financing of the NHI. Only by controlling quantity with price can we raise people's cost awareness of health care. We must tackle the overuse of health care together through communication with the medical profession and patients.

Drug Co-payments May Increase Slightly

The ceiling of the co-payment for drugs, which is currently NTD 200 may be raised slightly. The co-payment for examinations and tests, which were not collected before, may also be charged according to the level of medical institutions that perform the examinations and tests. The NHIA is also discussing restoring the co-payment for refillable drug prescriptions for chronic illnesses, and co-payment for those who have major illnesses.

The purpose of "increasing co-payment" is not to increase the financial income of the NHI but to reduce unnecessary medical behaviours of the people and doctors. When clinicians have more time to take care of patients, the quality of care will naturally improve. It also helps clinicians to earn reasonable rewards and prevents medical staff burnout.

Conclusion

A stable and sufficient source of insurance income is the cornerstone of the sustainable operation of the NHI. The actuarial calculations of the premium rate and financial estimation help to understand the future financial situation of the NHI and respond early.

The co-payment not only raises cost awareness of the insured when using the resources of the NHI but also realises the spirit of user charge. It can motivate people to seek proper care in a tiered healthcare system and achieve the goal of effective medical resource utilisation and sound financial security of the NHI.

The NHIA is committed to protecting the rights and interests of disadvantaged groups with proactive actions. We also look forward to seeking consensus through social dialogues and identify more disadvantaged groups in need of help. As everyone may get sick, it is the responsibility of the government to protect people's health effectively. By doing so, we can guarantee the appropriate distribution of medical resources and the sustainable development of the NHI. Let us work together for the sustainability of the NHI.

Reference

1. 20210111 健康名人堂, United Daily News.

Chapter 3
Payment Structure

**Yu-Pin Chang, Yu-Chuan Liu, Wen-Wen Chang, Chun-Fu Lee,
Chun-Mei Lin, Shu-Hwa Lin, and Min-Yu Lee**

Introduction

After medical institutions provide medical services to patients, the insurer—the National Health Insurance Administration (NHIA)—pays them through various measures constituting a "payment system." The various payment methods include fee-for-service, case payment, per diem payment, pay-for-performance, Taiwan diagnosis-related groups (Tw-DRGs), capitation payment (in the pilot program), and global budget payment (Fig. 3.1). Different payment systems influence how medical providers deliver medical services, which subsequently affects patient treatment and care. At the same time, they have a tremendous impact on the overall growth in medical expenses, the allocation of medical resources, and medical efficiency and quality. Therefore, how to choose a more appropriate payment system requires further discussion.

The payment system of health insurance in most countries is "fee-for-service," that is, the more you do to patients, the more money you make. The advantage is that the doctors can decide the treatment according to the disease severity, patient's need, and the volume of medical services provided is related to remuneration. The disadvantage is that the insurer pays strictly for the medical services the doctor provides with no consideration of treatment quality or efficacy, thus creating no incentives for medical providers to reduce the number of unnecessary medical services they provide.

Although the diversified payment methods have been implemented successfully, the "fee-for-service" is still the main payment method, which results in fast-growing medical expenses. In addition, the medical resources are limited, so the global

Y.-P. Chang (✉) · Y.-C. Liu · W.-W. Chang · C.-F. Lee · C.-M. Lin · S.-H. Lin · M.-Y. Lee
National Health Insurance Administration, Ministry of Health and Welfare, Taipei, Taiwan
e-mail: A110413@nhi.gov.tw; B111262@nhi.gov.tw; wenwen@nhi.gov.tw; chunfu@nhi.gov.tw; melin@nhi.gov.tw; F118001@nhi.gov.tw; plmy@nhi.gov.tw

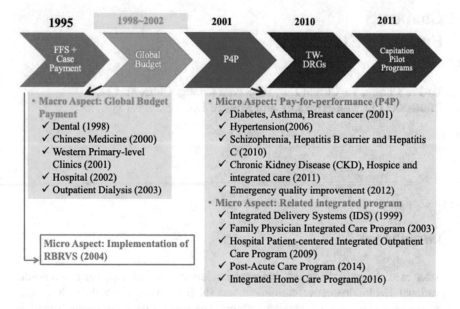

Fig. 3.1 Evolution of the National Health Insurance payment system

budget payment system was implemented in 2002 to promote reasonable use of medical resources and strike a balance of conflicting interests between payers and medical service providers under the negotiation mechanisms.

The National Health Insurance (NHI) Fee Schedule is adjusted from the macro and objective perspective to promote appropriate and high-quality medical behaviors. The NHIA constantly revises the fee schedule to encourage medical providers with reasonable medical payments and improve the current medical environment.

Different Payment Methods in the National Health Insurance System

A Simple Explanation of the Global Budget Payment System

In the global budget payment system, the payers and the medical service providers negotiate the total medical expenditure (global budget) in advance for certain medical services, including dental outpatient, Chinese medicine outpatient, Western medicine outpatient, and inpatient services for the future period (usually 1 year ahead) and reimburse the medical services provided by each medical department during the period. A payment system such as this is aimed at ensuring the financial balance of health insurance.

Taiwan's NHI global budget has "upper limit expenditure." The annual global budget for health insurance expenditures is allocated in advance based on the growth of the cost and the volume of medical services. The relative value units (RVUs) of medical services reflect the costs of those services, and the amount paid per RVU is retrospectively priced by dividing the actual total medical service volume (RVUs) into the global budget cap. When the actual total medical service volume is greater than the originally agreed-upon total medical service volume, the payment amount per RVU decreases, and conversely, if the total volume is less than the originally agreed-upon total, the payment amount per RVU increases. Because this payment system has a fixed annual global budget, the medical expenditures can be controlled precisely. Medical providers will be aware of the annual global budget in advance, so incentives to obtain excessive remuneration by providing excessive medical services can be reduced through peer constraints. Therefore, overall medical behaviors should be inclined toward a reasonable direction.

Introduction to Each Payment Method

1. Fee-for-service: the predominant payment method of the NHI. The RVUs of each medical service, drug, and medical device are set, and the medical providers submit the claim for medical expenses to the insurer based on the medical services they provide every month.
2. Pay-for-performance: quality-oriented payment systems are promoted for diseases with large cost impacts, many patients, and care models that need to be improved to encourage hospitals to establish a patient-centered integrated care model. This payment method provides additional incentives such as managed care fees and quality bonuses to encourage medical institutions to improve the quality of care. At present, the pay-for-performance plans for diabetes, asthma, breast cancer, schizophrenia, early-stage chronic kidney diseases and pre-end-stage renal disease, hepatitis B and C tracking, full-course maternity care, early intervention for developmental retardation, chronic obstructive pulmonary disease, and hospital medication safety improvement have been implemented.
3. Case payment: for relatively simple medical services with less variation in consumption, a fixed package payment is set for the medical visit—for example, delivery, cataract surgery, extracorporeal shock wave lithotripsy for urinary tract stones.
4. Tw-DRGs: diagnosis-related groups (DRGs) is an inpatient payment method that groups diseases with similar diagnostic categories or similar treatments and then subdivides them into different DRGs according to patient age, gender, comorbidities, complications, and discharge status. The RVUs of inpatient payment of each DRG service were calculated based on claims from previous years.
5. Per diem payment: for inpatient cases with specific diseases or specific treatments, the per diem payment is set according to the type of disease. Regardless of the number of medical services provided, the medical expenses are calculated

based on the length of stay at the hospital and the per diem payment, for example, chronic psychiatric inpatient, inpatient hospice.

6. Capitation payment: capitation is a prospective payment method that providers are paid in a fixed amount per patient, and the medical expenses are prearranged between the insurer and the medical providers based on the different health types of patients, for example, age, gender, medical cost. By building an integrated medical care system and emphasizing the concept of patient-centered care, preventive health care, acute and chronic disease care, and other health care are provided by specific medical providers for the comprehensive care.

The advantages and disadvantages of each payment system are described in Table 3.1.

Implementation of Pay-for-Performance and Bundled Payment in Recent Years

The promotion for the pay-for-performance payment method is carried out by several projects. The process indicators and the performance indicators are set in each project, and medical institutions receive additional rewards according to their implementation conditions. In 2019, the total RVUs of the implementation of pay-for-performance projects were 1.42 billion, and the implementation status is shown in Table 3.2.

In 2019, the number of case payment cases totaled 406,000, medical expenses totaled 9.84 billion RVUs, and the number of medical visits amounted to approximately 315,000, all showing an increasing trend year by year. In addition, the Tw-DRGs have been implemented under the NHI since 2010. A total of 401 DRGs were implemented in the first and second phases in January 2010 and July 2014 respectively. After the DRG reclassification in 2020, a total of 407 DRGs have been implemented. In 2019, the medical expenses of DRGs accounted for 18% of the overall inpatient medical expenses.

Global Budget Payment System

Because the global budget is negotiated by payers and medical providers through the platform of the National Health Insurance Committee (NHIC), in theory, various cost factors have been fully considered. As a consensus on the budget has been reached (or directly approved by the health authority without a consensus), providers have to reach professional consensus among their peers by exercising strategies such as file or data analysis, resource sharing to reduce medical service volume and increase the RVU value and eventually avoid falling into a vicious circle of doing more and receiving less.

Table 3.1 Comparison of the advantages and disadvantages of various payment methods

Payment method	Advantages	Disadvantages
Fee-for-service	1. Simple administration 2. Medical services are provided based on clinical judgment 3. High acceptability to medical service providers because of the low financial risk	1. It probably induces unnecessary medical services, including medical tests, examinations, medication or surgery, because medical service providers lack incentives to make the best use of medical resources 2. Financial risks are mainly borne by the insurer
Pay-for-performance	1. Encourages medical service providers to deliver high-quality medical services through an incentive mechanism 2. High-quality medical services and care to reduce subsequent medical expenses or complications	1. Medical care quality is difficult to measure 2. Administrative cost of medical care is high
Case payment	Encourages medical service providers to actively control costs and reduce unnecessary medical services	1. Only apply to simple diseases, the benefits of comprehensive management are limited. 2. The severity of the patient's illness may increase the medical service providers' financial risk
Taiwan diagnosis-related groups (Tw-DRGs)	1. Encourages medical service providers to actively control costs and reduce unnecessary medical services 2. Strengthens the clinical guideline and pathway management, standardizes treatment procedures, and improves healthcare quality and efficiency 3. Can be used as a tool to compare quality	1. The severity and the complexity of the patient's illness may increase the medical service providers' financial risk 2. Whether the statistic of the consumption of medical resources and the classification of clinical diseases are reasonable is worth further discussion 3. May cause medical institutions to reduce necessary medical services or patients to be discharged prematurely
Per diem payment	1. Simple administration 2. Reduces unnecessary medical services	1. Only applicable to a few inpatient cases 2. Not taking the severity of the patients into consideration, so the medical service providers tend to treat patients with mild illness or extend inpatient days
Capitation payment	Incentivizes medical service providers to provide fully responsible and efficient medical services and healthcare for people in the community	1. Owing to the dynamicity of the health status, it is difficult to determine the medical expenses required by people with different health statuses. If the risk adjustment is not comprehensive, medical institutions may tend to choose healthy insured individuals 2. The accessibility to medical care is high, and it is difficult for a single medical institution to provide comprehensive care

Table 3.2 The implementation of various pay-for-performance projects in 2019

Project/global budget sector	Clinics				Hospitals			
	No. of institutions	Million RVUs	Cases	Care rate	No. of institutions	Million RVUs	Cases	Care rate
Diabetes	909	328.6	246,940	42.1%	273	691.2	539,679	60.0%
Asthma	576	44.8	81,814	38.6%	142	44.7	53,983	25.4%
Breast cancer	–	–	–	–	5	75.4	11,164	7.3%
Schizophrenia	18	1.2	1628	10.5%	125	53	59,668	74.0%
Hepatitis B and C tracking	363	14.7	80,368	41.5%	198	34.2	187,763	39.5%
Full-course maternity care	29	12.1	9705	21.2%	92	61.5	44,659	38.0%
Early treatment for development retardation	3	0.4	114	8.3%	24	3.7	1383	11.9%
Chronic obstructive pulmonary disease	90	0.9	1406	38.1%	130	25.6	20,471	35.2%
Hospital medication safety improvement	–	–	–	–	103	27.9	40,953	–

Note:
1. Cases: the cases were actually claimed under the project among all inpatient and outpatient claims in 2019
2. Care rate: the numerator is the number of the cases actually claimed under the project among all inpatient and outpatient claims in 2019; the denominator is the number of cases claimed under the project with a specified diagnosis code

Planning the Annual Global Budget

As the global budget is determined in advance, the negotiating procedure for the annual global budget occurs before the beginning of the year. The health authority—the Ministry of Health and Welfare (MOHW), taking into account the country's overall economic development and the medical needs of the people, drafts the global budget range for the next year. After consulting the NHIC, the drafted global budget will be submitted to the Executive Yuan for approval 6 months before the start of the year. Then the NHIC, which is composed of representatives of the insured, employers, medical institutions, experts, and scholars, is responsible for the negotiation (Fig. 3.2).

Taking the global budget in 2021, for instance, the MOHW suggested that the range of global budget growth rate in 2021 should be 2.907–5.0% after comprehensively considering factors such as overall population growth, aging, medical service costs, new drugs, and special medical devices, allocation of medical resources, and healthcare quality. After being submitted to the Executive Yuan for reconsideration,

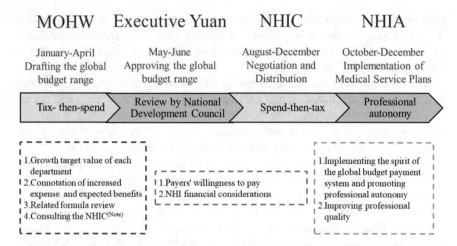

Fig. 3.2 Procedure for negotiating the annual global budget
Note: According to Article 60 of the National Health Insurance Act, the annual global budget of medical expenses shall be drafted by the health authority and submitted to the Executive Yuan for approval after consulting the NHIC

the range was approved to be 2.907–4.5% and transferred to the NHIC for negotiation. Eventually, the global budget growth rate for 2021 announced was 4.107%, and the global budget was New Taiwan dollars (NTD) 783.6 billion.

The global budget is allocated quarterly, which means the payment amount per RVU is retrospectively settled after the end of the quarter, so the situation that the budget is used up before the end of the year will not happen.

Global Budget Distribution and Management

Taiwan's National Health Insurance Act (hereinafter referred to as the NHI Act), which stipulates the implementation of the global budget payment system, the global budget of dental outpatients, Chinese medicine outpatients, Western primary-level clinics, hospitals, and other budgets (not covered by the global budget of the four departments mentioned above and the cross-departmental budget), was implemented since July 1998, July 2000, July 2001, and July 2002 respectively. Therefore, it can be said that Taiwan has fully implemented the global budget payment system since July 2002.

Moreover, to promote the balanced medical resource allocations, the principle of "the budget follows the people" is used when distributing the budget to the six districts to strengthen the financial and healthcare responsibilities of each district. For example, in the first year when the global budget of dental outpatients was implemented, 10% of the global budget was distributed according to the adjusted "population risk" of each district and 90% was distributed according to the actual proportion of medical expenses for beneficiaries in each district in the year before the global budget of dental outpatients was implemented. In 2007, the budget distribution was 100% based on the number of those insured and adjusted according to the "population risk" of each district.

The distribution of the global budget of each department and the regional budgets are macrolevel strategies, and microlevel supporting measures are still necessary to improve the efficiency of medical services and reduce medical waste, for example, active investigation and punishment with violations, payment system reforms, fee schedule adjustment, motivation for effective medical services, review system improvement, information system upgrade, enhanced peer management among the medical profession, promotion of My Health Bank system.

The annual global budget is the result of the negotiation and mutual understanding between the payers and the medical providers. Every dollar of the global budget also comes from the premiums paid by those insured, so it must be spent in a worthy way to buy necessary medical care. Medical waste is the last thing we want to see. Therefore, purchasing medical care of higher efficiency and better quality through the improvement of the payment system is the overall goal of the insurer.

Reducing the Provision of Unnecessary and Excessive Medical Services to Increase the Value of the Relative Value Unit

The COVID-19 pandemic has caused a significant decrease in the number of medical visits in 2020. The number of outpatient visits was 360 million in 2018 and increased to 368 million in 2019. Instead of increasing continuously, the number of outpatient visits decreased to 340 million in 2020, which was 28 million less than the number in 2019 and 20 million less than the number in 2018 (Fig. 3.3). During this period, there were no major changes in people's health.

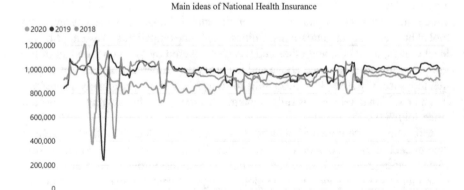

Fig. 3.3 Weekly moving average of outpatient visits (full calendar year 2018 vs. 2019 vs. 2020)

Because the global budget has been fixed, the reduction in the number of medical visits does not reduce the income of the medical institutions from the NHI global budget. On the contrary, owing to the increase in the RVU value, doctors can get the same amount of income as before, without seeing as many patients and this is the path that we have been following. Doctors can concentrate on treating patients properly instead of making reparative appointments and providing more and more medical services to create potential RVUs. This concept was verified during the pandemic. According to the preliminary settlement results of the global budget, the RVU value of the primary-level Western clinics in 2020 is expected to reach more than NTD 1 per RVU.

Relative Value Units and Relative Value Unit Values are the Overall Causes and Outcomes of Each Other

Generally speaking, there is a 7–9% gap between the claimed RVUs and the global budget (Fig. 3.4). Even when only taking the approved RVUs into consideration, there is still a gap of 2–4% from the global budget. According to the RVU growth trend of outpatients and inpatients (Fig. 3.5), the growth rate of outpatient RVUs is higher than that of inpatients, and the percentage of outpatient RVUs reached almost 70% in 2019. With further analysis of outpatient RVUs, the growth rate of medication costs and diagnostic and treatment costs (including examination and test costs) is higher.

Some doctors complain that the RVUs for certain items are too low, but the RVU values often drop after the RVUs increase. Some doctors are not satisfied with the low RVU value, hoping to fix the RVU value of certain medical specialties, diseases, or treatments within a certain range. However, with a limited global budget, when the RVU values of these items are guaranteed, the RVU values of other items inevitably drop. The dilemma of whether to raise the payment of certain items or to guarantee their RVU value and fairly satisfy providers' requests is indeed a difficult problem to address.

To promote the tiered medical care and encourage large hospitals to transfer stable chronic outpatients to primary medical institutions, it is necessary to relatively increase the payment of emergency and critical care to large hospitals. After patients are transferred to the primary medical institutions, it is also crucial to enhance the capability of primary care providers with appropriate payment to maintain the patient's confidence in seeking medical care from them continuously. Both of these goals could be effectively attained by increasing the RVU and guaranteeing the RVU value.

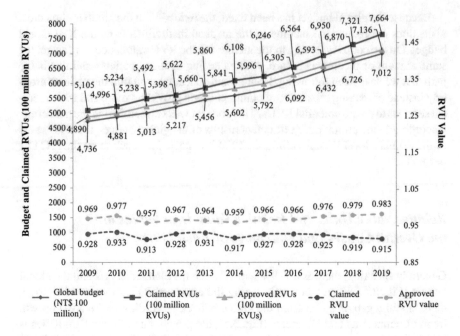

Fig. 3.4 The difference between the global budget and the claimed and approved relevant value units (RVUs) from 2009 to 2019
Note:
1. Global budget (blue), approved RVUs (green), and claimed RVUs (red), excluding other departments
2. Approved RVU value: global budget/approved RVUs (green)
3. Claimed RVU value: global budget/claimed RVUs (red)

Adjusting Relative Value Units to Promote Balanced Development of Medical Specialties

After the implementation of a global budget payment system, each medical treatment was related to a corresponding payment of RVUs. However, the medical environment has changed since the NHI system was launched 27 years ago. The cost of treatments related to emergency and critical care has risen rapidly, so the relevant payment also needs to be modified accordingly. To avoid uneven development among the medical specialties, the NHIA has actively striven for budgets to universally increase the payment for main departments such as internal medicine, surgery, obstetrics and gynecology, and pediatrics in recent years.

Over the past 3 years, a budget of NTD 19.5 billion was allocated to adjust the payment for Western medicine, including:

1. In 2017, NTD 11 billion was invested to increase the RVUs of emergency and critical care, including the markup rate of ward fees of district hospitals, inpatient nursing fees, and outpatient diagnostic fees; the first-stage outpatient diagnostic fees in primary medical institutions were increased by 20 RVUs.

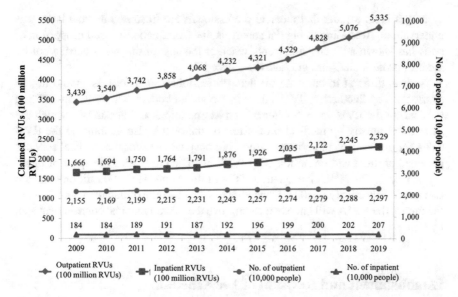

Fig. 3.5 Trends in the number of outpatient and inpatient claimed relevant value units (excluding other departments) and the number of the patient population from 2009 to 2019

2. In 2018, NTD 3.1 billion was invested to increase 5% of the inpatient nursing fees for the intensive care unit (ICU), 31% of the CPR payment, and 20% of the payment in 10 items, including simple sutures/dressing changes, and to encourage district hospitals to provide medical services on holidays.
3. In 2019, NTD 5.4 billion was allocated to increase payment for 116 items of emergency and critical care (with a 4–80% adjustment), and 278 items of operations or treatments that had either not been adjusted or were only adjusted fewer than twice in past years (with a 20% adjustment). In addition to modifying the anesthesia fees as an enhanced markup item for pediatric patients, the inpatient nursing fees for acute general ward and inpatient diagnostic fees were also increased by 3% and 13.5% respectively; a 20% markup for caring for people aged over 75, a 10% markup for outpatient diagnostic fees at night in district hospitals, and a 50% markup for emergency diagnostic fees by specialist physicians were added; the first-stage outpatient diagnostic fees in primary medical institutions were increased by 6 RVUs.

Guaranteeing the Relative Value Unit Value to Encourage Investment in the Healthcare Workforce

Human resources is the most valuable asset of healthcare facilities. However, medical professionals often complain that they have worked hard without getting the "affirmation" they deserve. Because the RVU value for medical professionals' labor or machine output fluctuates in the same way under the NHI global budget payment system, it is no wonder that medical professionals are frustrated by how labor was undervalued. According to big data analysis, the examination-related proportion of costs has shown an increasing trend, whereas the cost of diagnosis carried out by medical professionals has gradually decreased.

As it is difficult to cultivate medical professionals, their efforts should not be overlooked by fluctuating RVU values in the global budget. Therefore, in addition to securing the RVU value for items such as operations and anesthesia, which are carried out mostly by medical professionals, the NHIA also guaranteed the RVU value for emergency and critical care in big hospitals and for the medical services provided at night and on holidays by small hospitals to realize the spirit of tiered medical care. The NHIA has secured NTD 1 billion and NTD 500 million for these two items respectively in 2021. Depending on the outcome of budget negotiation, in the future, the NHIA will endeavor to improve the overall medical environment step by step.

Establishment and Revision of Fee Schedule

After clinical medical professionals provide patients with medical services such as diagnoses, examinations and tests, treatment, surgery, and anesthesia, they are paid according to the "NHI Fee Schedule and Reference List for Medical Services" (hereinafter referred to as the Fee Schedule) by submitting a claim for medical costs to the NHIA under the categories of Western medicine, dental services, Chinese medicine, home care, psychiatric community rehabilitation, case payment, etc. The NHIA has continued to allocate budget for expansion and revision of treatment items to further reflect technological progress, clinical needs, and reasonable rewards for health professionals. At present, nearly 4,600 medical service items are included.

Fee Schedule Revision Procedure

Because the revision of the fee schedule involves the cost of medical institutions and the clinical practice considerations such as the efficacy, safety, and technical proficiency of each diagnosis or treatment, most revision proposals were submitted to the NHIA by medical institutions or related medical specialist associations. The application form includes Chinese and English names of new items, main clinical function and objectives, comparison with traditional diagnosis or treatment, estimated performing volume and NHI financial impact assessment; report with evidence-based data, cost analysis tables, operating procedures (including the number of hours invested by various medical professionals in each process) and supporting documents should also be submitted. After collecting relevant information and opinions from clinical professionals, and conducting comprehensive assessment,

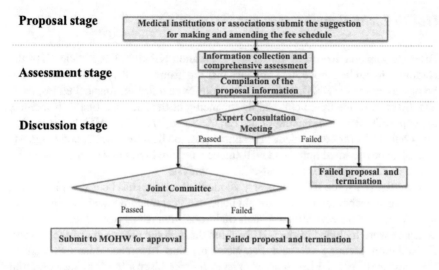

Proposal stage

Assessment stage

Discussion stage

Fig. 3.6 Fee schedule revision procedure

Table 3.3 Fee schedule revision process

	Administrative review stage	Professional review stage	Discussion stage
Proposing entity	Submission and resubmission according NHIA's review result		
NHIA	Replying to the proposing entity for correction or additional documents	1. Replying to the proposing entity that the proposal will be submitted to an expert consultation meeting 2. Drafting review opinions and asking for professional opinions 3. Investigating out-of-pocket prices 4. Searching for international situation of payment 5. Confirming the inclusion of priced medical devices or drugs	1. Arranging meeting agenda 2. Submitting to Expert Consultation Meeting 3. Submitting to Joint Committee
External expert		Completing the review opinion form	Discussion in the meeting

the NHIA submits proposals to the "Expert Consultation Meeting on NHI Fee Schedule and Reference List for Medical Services" for approval, and then to the "NHI Fee Schedule and Reference List for Medical Services Joint Committee" for discussion. After the members of the committee agree on whether to include an individual item in the benefits of the NHI, the NHIA submits the agreed items to the MOHW, which announces the effectiveness of the inclusions. The complete procedure and process are shown in Fig. 3.6 and Table 3.3.

Health Technology Assessment

After the implementation of the second-generation NHI in 2013, Article 42 of the National Health Insurance Act stipulates that the insurer shall adapt the health technology assessment (HTA), and shall consider human health, medical ethics, cost-effectiveness of the treatment, and the financing of the National Health Insurance, to support the decision-making of the NHIA. Since 2013, the NHIA has started to carry out HTAs for costly medical technologies, medical treatments, and diagnosis items that have a large impact on NHI finance, require literature confirmation on its efficacy or in-depth domestic cost-effective analysis.

Over the years, the HTAs of nearly 40 medical services has been completed, and new medical technologies that brought better medical outcomes and were proven to be safer and more cost-effective than traditional treatments according to relevant evidence were included in the NHI benefits through the discussion of the "Expert Consultation Meeting on NHI Fee Schedule and Reference List for Medical Services" and the "NHI Fee Schedule and Reference List for Medical Services Joint Committee." In total, five items are covered by the NHI currently, including "transcatheter insertion or replacement of permanent leadless pacemaker," "molecular adsorbent recirculating system," "vagus nerve stimulation," "transcatheter aortic valve implantation," and "bipolar transurethral resection/plasma vaporization of the prostate." In addition, the surgical fees for "Da Vinci radical prostatectomy" and "Da Vinci robotic partial nephrectomy" are covered by the NHI as existing items (such as laparoscopy), whereas the medical devices remain out-of-pocket items.

The HTAs will continue to be conducted to support the decision-making on NHI payments. Furthermore, the NHIA will introduce "Health Technology Reassessment" for follow-up surveillance of the performance of diagnosis and treatment covered to ensure the quality of medical care and NHI financial stability.

Items Not Been Covered by the NHI

According to the fee schedule, when the NHI-contracted medical institutions provide medical services not listed in the fee schedule, they should submit the claim based on the RVUs of the most similar items in the relevant category. Therefore, when a medical institution carries out a treatment or diagnosis not covered by the NHI, it should claim the reimbursement following the corresponding table listed in the "Claiming Standards of Items Not Listed in the Fee Schedule for the Contracted Medical Institutions" published on the NHIA's official website. For example, "left atrial appendage occlusion" should be claimed according to the current code 68005B "Cardiorrhaphy for heart wound or injury." As for other items that are not listed in the corresponding table, they should be claimed by the medical institutions as the most similar items in the relevant category of the fee schedule.

In addition, when people seek medical care and receive medical treatment not covered by the NHI, except for the out-of-pocket items, the rest of the items that are already covered are still paid by the NHIA. For example, when people seek medical care owing to illness and agree to receive the out-of-pocket "high-intensity focused ultrasound" operation, except for the out-of-pocket costs of the operation and related medical consumables, other inpatient costs during this hospital stay (including consultation fees, ward fees, examination fees, medicine fees, anesthesia fees, etc.) can be claimed via the NHIA. As for the necessity or appropriateness of the surgical treatment, it should be determined by their professional judgment and will be reviewed by medical experts of the NHIA.

Self-Management Plan Under the Global Budget Payment System and Corresponding Measures of Insufficient Budgeting

Since its inception in 1995, the NHI inherited the payment system of the Government Employees' Health Insurance and Labor Insurance, which reimburse medical expenses mainly in the "fee-for-service" system and supplemented by "case payment." On the basis of fee-for-service, the overall medical expenditure has increased significantly from NTD 143.3 billion in the first year of the NHI to NTD 268.7 billion in 1998, which is almost doubled in just 4 years. Therefore, the NHIA has learned from developed countries such as Canada, Germany, and Australia, and implemented the global budget payment system in the dentist department in 1998. The global budget payment system was applied to the traditional Chinese medicine department and Western medicine clinics subsequently, as well as the hospital department in July 2002. The annual NHI medical expenses are negotiated and determined by the government, payers, experts, scholars, and medical service providers. The overall medical expenditure in 2020 has reached NTD 752.6 billion, a growth of 5.25 times in 25 years. After the implementation of the global budget payment system, when the growth of the global budget is less than that of the medical service volume, the value of each RVU is less than NTD 1, which means that the payment is the discounted. The medical professionals have often discussed this situation.

Self-Management Plan

In order to allocate the limited global budget appropriately, the NHIA optimizes the returned deducted medical reimbursement from abnormal cases for hospitals to reuse. Each division of the NHIA also establishes a co-management mechanism with hospital representatives within its jurisdiction to negotiate and formulate a "self-management plan," which encompasses various cost control and quality assurance measures.

Subtracting Relative Value Units Directly

The NHIA divisions set the "target value of the RVU" through the abovementioned co-management mechanism and allocate the "hospital-specific global budget" to each hospital in advance. The NHIA divisions provide review exemption as an incentive for those hospitals that do not exceed the allocated quota to encourage self-management, hoping to avoid the devaluation of RVUs attributed to the significant growth in medical services. If the RVUs of medical services exceed the allocated quota, the excess will be subtracted directly or via a sampling rate in proportion with excess RVUs.

Sharing the Relative Value Unit Gap

Some divisions of the NHIA estimate the value of the RVU at the end of the quarter. If the estimated value of the RVU cannot reach the preset "target RVU value," the differences between them will be shared by all hospitals. After negotiating special items (such as rare diseases, hemophilia, or anti-rejection medication after organ transplantation) and items that require guaranteed values, the hospitals share the gap of RVUs according to the "percentage of contribution to RVU growth" and "proportion of expenses," so that the value of the RVU can reach the target. In this way, each hospital claims with the better priced RVUs to acquire reallocated medical expenses.

Analysis and Reflections

It has been more than 27 years since the implementation of the NHI. People in Taiwan have a high level of freedom in seeking medical care, and the expectation of receiving high-quality service with low payment is so deeply rooted that controlling the volume of medical services is quite difficult. In the past 20 years, the average RVU value in the hospital department has always been less than NTD 1 (Fig. 3.7).

The operation methods of each NHIA division are introduced as follows:

1. NHIA: Taipei Division

Taking the NHIA-Taipei Division (the largest division, which includes Taipei, New Taipei, Keelung, Yilan, Kinmen, and Lianjiang's six counties and cities) as an example, the annual difference between budget and claimed RVUs is as high as NTD 19.2 billion if the value of one RVU equates to NTD 1 in the past 5 years (Fig. 3.8). Using the aforementioned measures such as self-management, RVU subtraction, and RVU gap sharing, the Taipei Division barely maintains the value of one RVU to be higher than NTD 0.9. However, it is difficult to remunerate hospitals properly for the medical services they provide. This so-called "sweat hospital" phenomenon indicates the room for improvement in management measures.

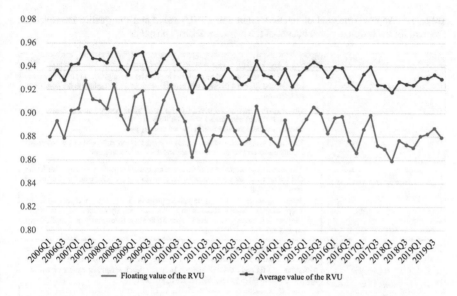

Fig. 3.7 The relative value unit value of global budget for hospitals from 2006 to 2019

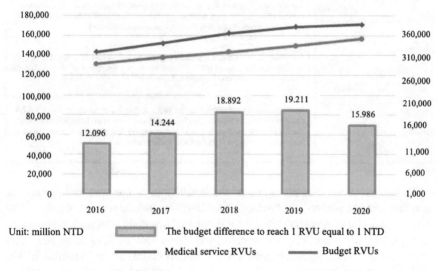

Fig. 3.8 The relative value units claimed, budget, and difference in the NHIA Taipei Division (medical treatment business group)

2. NHIA: Northern Division

The approval process of RVU value and the quality improvement program for the global budget of the Northern District hospitals is described in Table 3.4.

3. NHIA: Central Division

Table 3.4 Approval process of relative value unit (RVU) value and the quality improvement program for the hospital global budget of the Northern District hospitals

Implementation process	Description
Planning and explanation of the RVU value and the quality improvement program for the hospital global budget	1. The program next year will be discussed in pre-brief meetings held in November every year, and the Northern Division will compile opinions from hospitals in the jurisdiction for reference 2. The program planning and content of the RVU value and the quality improvement program for the hospital global budget for the next year will be discussed in co-management, a meeting held in December every year 3. The dean's symposium and the hospital briefing are held at the end of December and January each year to explain the content and details of the program
Selection of the global budget program and contract signing	1. The program and the planning of the RVUs are completed in early January of each year, and the hospitals are informed about the program and the basic target RVUs after the hospital briefing 2. Each hospital chooses to participate in program A or program B and signs the supplementary contract according to its decision will. By default, hospitals choose program B if no reply is received before the deadline (late January to early February every year)
The quarterly expense claim, review, and approval	The quarterly expense claim, review, and approval are implemented according to the "National Health Insurance Medical Expense Claims and Payment and Review Measures of Medical Service" and the program. Each hospital's expenses will be approved within 60 days after claims are completed
The adjustment mechanism for allocation and approval of target RVUs in the global budget	According to the global budget settlement schedule and the content of the program, the adjustment mechanism for allocation and approval of target RVUs is applied quarterly (early March, June, September, and December) to reward improved quality, encouraged policy compliance, and the excess reward (quality indicators, increase in number of patients seeking medical care, increase in amount of medical services of acute disease provided, severe disease, cancer, and childbirth)
Approval of the program, expenses recovery, and subtraction	According to the result of adjusted allocation and approval of the target RVUs, the RVU claims that exceed the target will be directly subtracted in plan A, and the differences between actual claims and targets will be shared in plan B
Approval of the global budget program and follow-up	Hospitals that do not claim over the target RVUs: They can apply for retrial for cases deleted by the reviewer; for hospitals that claim over the target RVUs already, the NHIA will conduct inspections if suspected and give the review opinions feedback to the hospitals and counsel for improvement.

To safeguard the medical rights of the inhabitants of the area and protect the development of hospitals, the NHIA Central Division ensures reimbursement of five specific items by setting target RVUs for individual hospitals or overall quotas in the management program. The abovementioned items include long-term respirator usage management program, hospitals with quarterly claims under 36 million RVUs, RVUs for emergency triage classification level 1 or 2 and hospital stay for major trauma or cancer surgery, drug fee for outpatient and inpatient cancer chemotherapy, and single outpatient prescription for catastrophic illness with drug fee greater than 6000 RVUs. The Central Division refers to the original claim value of hospitals and peer claim value when formulating relevant management and control programs.

To prevent waste of medical resources while attaining service quality and rationality, the Central Division uses the unit price for outpatient and inpatient drug fees and nondrug fees as monitoring indicators. In addition, the quality indicators are integrated into the reward mechanism to improve the care quality of hospitals.

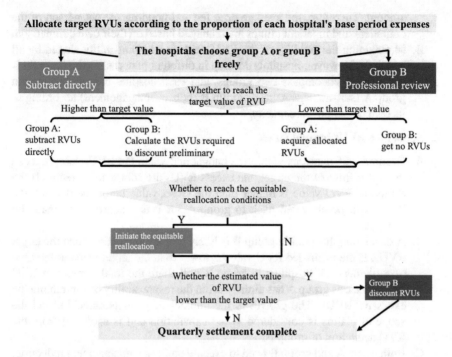

Fig. 3.9 Risk control and quality improvement program implementation framework of the hospital global budget relative value unit value in the NHIA Southern Division

4. NHIA: Southern Division

The management methods of the NHIA Southern Division include "allocation in advance," which means one's voluntary compliance with the rules and "supervision afterward," which means one's compliance with the rules under others' supervision. The "Risk Control and Quality Improvement Plan of the Hospital Global Budget RVU Value of the NHIA Southern Division" is a kind of allocation in advance, which encourages self-management of hospitals by setting a "hospital-specific global budget." The overall execution structure is shown in Fig. 3.9 and described as follows:

1. The "hospital-specific global budget" and select a group

   A. According to the available budget and the target value of the RVU negotiated by the medical professionals, the Southern Division acquired the total number of RVUs to allocate. Then the "hospital-specific global budget" is formulated based on the proportion of each hospital's base period and the composition of providers (the number of medical personnel). This is a kind of quantity management. As the medical expenses consist of price and quantity, the Southern Division must also control the unit price as well as the total amount. Therefore, the average drug fee and nondrug fee per person of the outpatient and inpatient clinics are managed based on their own comparison.

B. Maintaining the stability of the RVU value is a responsibility shared by all hospitals. However, hospitals develop in different patterns, so the program is designed to encompass two groups, and each hospital can choose to join group A (self-management) or group B (nonself-management) according to its own development capacity.

2. Deduct the RVUs beyond target

A. Group A self-manages within the budget and when the RVU claims exceed the upper limit of the target, the excess RVUs are subtracted directly. If the estimated RVU value is higher than the target value before settlement, the RVUs will be allocated back to group A for it is a contribution made by group A.

B. A developing hospital in group B is likely to file more claims than the target RVUs. If the estimated RVU value is lower than the target value at the time of settlement, all hospitals in group B will share the total number of RVU differences, as group A has already taken the responsibility of subtracting the excessive RVUs. The growth in the number of patients cared for and the scope of claims is considered in the calculation and is excluded from the RVU deduction of group B.

C. Both group A and group B need to execute unit price management reduction. In quarterly settlements, group A reduces RVUs down to the upper limit target as it already has a direct subtraction mechanism, and the insufficient part will be directly deducted from the target RVUs for the next year. As for group B, RVUs are reduced in the current quarter.

3. Redistribute equitably after weighting cost growth rate in the two groups

A. To balance the responsibility of caring for the patients in these two groups, the Southern Division weighted the difference between the growth rate of the service volume and the supply volume of the two groups before settlement. When one group has much more growth rate than the other one, the budget would be redistributed to the other group to limit the difference of growth rate within 3%. The purpose is to prevent group A from reducing the provision of medical care owing to the financial risk, to ensure the well-being of patients, curb the buck passing, and prevent drastic differences in the net growth rate between the two groups.

Although the Global Budget Payment System of the NHI can control the growth of national medical expenses, competition can easily occur among medical institutions, as the payment is based on the fee-for-service model. To prevent the interference of uncertain or low RVU values with hospital operations, all NHIA divisions adjust expenses according to their income and execute programs to stabilize the RVU values of the hospital global budget. The related implementation strategy is commonly known as the "hospital self-management plan."

5. NHIA: Kaoping Division

The NHIA Kaoping Division provides information feedback to contracted institutions, intending to strengthen the management of institutions and reduce the medical waste. The NHIA understands that the medical RVUs would lead to medical waste and thus, it is necessary to continuously develop various global budget management strategies. The NHIA provides information from the National Health Insurance MediCloud System for medical institutions to inquire about patients' medical treatment records across different hospitals and clinics. In addition, it can assist physicians in obtaining a thorough understanding of past test/examination results and the drug use status of patients. This system benefits physicians in making relatively more precise diagnoses and prescriptions while reducing the waste of medical resources due to repetitive prescriptions or repetitive examinations/tests. The NHIA also provides personal health information through My Health Bank system so that the public can strengthen self-health management, identify illegal behaviors of institutions and physicians via big data analysis, and promote self-improvement through information disclosure and feedback, which facilitates professional communication among peers while conducting precise reviews.

6. NHIA: Eastern Division

The structure of the "Professional Review for Hospital Global Budget in the Eastern Division" is based on the number of hospital management targets, the number of claims, and hospital income in the same period last year. The NHIA Eastern Division also calculates the number of quarterly management targets in each hospital with multiple adjustment factors such as adjustment of the RVU growth rate of medical expenses for outpatient, inpatient, emergency and critical care, and the number of patients. If the hospital controls the RVUs within the target, or agrees with subtracting the excessive part directly, then it is regarded as a self-management (A-level) hospital, which is exempt from random sampling reviews. A hospital that chooses to be a nonself-management (non-A-level) hospital will have to share the RVU gap when the estimated RVU value in the jurisdiction is lower than 92% of the target value. The Eastern Division has included the mechanism of the RVU gap sharing in the program since 2008 and executed it until now (the gap-sharing mechanism is activated if the estimated value is higher than 0.92 before settlement). Owing to the impact of the epidemic in 2020, the target RVU value in the Eastern Division is estimated with a floating formula, and the upper and lower limits are set at 0.92–0.96, whereas the range of 2021 is 0.92–0.94.

As the population risk factor and the referral percentage were used to adjust the allocation of the hospital global budget in 2017, the annual budget of the Eastern Division was reduced. Through unremitting efforts, the Eastern Division has been awarded the risk transfer fund since 2019 and set the principles for the use of the risk transfer fund with the hospitals in the jurisdiction jointly. To look after the disadvantaged and support remote areas, the NHIA East Division used more than 70% of the risk transfer fund for various projects, such as the diabetes care plan, hepatitis C, cancer, emergency medicine, remote wound care, and others; the rest of the budget was included in the target management allocation to compensate for the increased medical expenses of each program.

The complaints about self-management of the hospital global budget from the medical community are inevitable, and this is a plight that both the medical community and the NHIA are facing. The insufficient budget will certainly not only affect the medical service for patients, but will even affect the overall development of the country's medical and related industries. For example, how will the value of the RVU respond to emergencies such as natural disasters, major accidents, or emerging infectious diseases? Besides supervising and balancing, payer representatives should face the concept of user fees squarely. Adjusting co-payment for the general public while protecting the economically disadvantaged may be a reform direction for the NHI.

Chapter 4
Comprehensive Policies

Po-Chang Lee, Yu-Pin Chang, and Yu-Yun Tung

Introduction

The National Health Insurance (NHI) is the most important cornerstone of social security, and the National Health Insurance Administration (NHIA) is always committed to providing comprehensive and continuous services for the insured. With the sharply escalating medical expenses, expenditure reduction and high-value health care is the only answer to protecting patients' medical rights with the limited resources that we have in hand. The NHIA has also implemented a number of programs for the medical needs of the super-aged society that Taiwan will face in the future.

Taiwan followed the steps of many advanced countries in separating medicine and pharmacy to realize pharmacists' role of integrating and reviewing prescriptions issued by physicians. The NHIA has endeavored to promote two-way referrals in the tiered medical care structure since 2017. We hope to improve the efficiency of the overall healthcare system by the redistribution of the workload and cooperation between hospitals at different levels. Therefore, in addition to a reimbursement increase for hospitalization and emergency treatment, differences in co-payment for referral visit from a different level of hospital was applied to encourage better healthcare-seeking behavior. Recently, co-payment adjustment was proposed to raise the public's cost awareness and address overuse.

P.-C. Lee (✉) · Y.-P. Chang · Y.-Y. Tung
National Health Insurance Administration, Ministry of Health and Welfare, Taipei, Taiwan
e-mail: pochang@nhi.gov.tw; A110413@nhi.gov.tw; A110935@nhi.gov.tw

P.-C. Lee et al. (eds.), *Digital Health Care in Taiwan*,
https://doi.org/10.1007/978-3-031-05160-9_4

Implementation of the Separation of Medicine and Pharmacy from a National Health Insurance Perspective[1]

Since the inception of the NHI in March 1995, improved access to the contracted medical institutions facilitated a great opportunity to implement an independent pharmaceutical service through the NHI system. Therefore, the pharmacist association advocated for the enactment of Article 102, Item 2 of the Pharmaceutical Affairs Act, to separate drug prescribing and dispensing. The clause mandated that after 2 years of implementation of the NHI, physicians can dispense drugs by themselves based on their own prescriptions only in the remote areas where practicing pharmaceutical personnel are not available or in the case of urgent need for medical treatment services. It became the legal basis for the independent pharmaceutical service.

The medical profession is quite dissatisfied with the amendment, feeling deprived of their right to dispense, so physicians and pharmacists hit the street separately to protest against the new policy. The separation of prescribing and dispensing not only eliminates the medical institutions' benefits derived from drug price differences but also causes hidden worries such as license leasing, fewer medicines than the hospitals, dispensing alternative drugs, and modifying prescriptions.

Because of the stalemate between medical and pharmaceutical professionals over the issue of separating medicine and pharmacy, the former Department of Health, Executive Yuan, adjusted the original single-track system[2] to a dual-track system. In this way, the physicians in the medical institutions can release prescriptions, or hire pharmacists to dispense the prescription in-house. In this controversial adjustment, clinical pharmacists become employees hired by physicians to dispense drugs. As there is an employment relationship, the intention of holding pharmacists accountable for the supervision and professional review of the prescription by separating medicine and pharmacy is easily weakened or even disappears. Owing to the implementation of the dual-track system, instead of practicing completely separately, most of the time medical and pharmaceutical professionals only cooperate to share the workload.

The NHIA was tasked to establish a system that incentivizes physicians to release prescriptions. Therefore, the NHIA paid an additional 25 relative value units (RVUs) for the prescription released by clinics and provided pharmacies with higher dispensing and drug fees, so that the pharmacy could earn an extra 51 RVUs[3] on each

---

[1] Taiwan Bar Journal.

[2] The single-track system is also known as the ideal division of professions. In addition to the division between the medical and pharmaceutical professions, the industries must also divide substantively. The property rights of the practice between the physician and the pharmacist must be independent, and there should be no overlap or conflict of practice interests. That is, pharmacists cannot be employed in pharmacies funded by physicians or in joint ventures between physicians and pharmacists.

[3] The payment for each prescription is different by 51 RVUs in a clinic or a pharmacy. Liberty Times, 10 January 2005.

prescription on average. But the payment incentive results in the peculiar phenomenon of "front-door pharmacy," which triggered the NHIA to monitor "unreasonable prescription release patterns from clinics": the NHIA would refuse to reimburse additional diagnosis fees for clinics that release more than 900 prescriptions or over 70% of its prescriptions to a designated pharmacy, and this pharmacy dispenses more than 70% of the prescriptions released from one clinic at the same time. However, the phenomenon of registering an individual pharmacy within the proximity of the clinics was not fully curbed until the NHIA completely canceled the payment for releasing prescriptions in July 2006 and simultaneously increased the payment for drug dispensing from 21 to 28 RVUs provided by the physician-hired pharmacist.

The Meaning of Separating Medicine and Pharmacy

The purpose of separating medicine and pharmacy is not only to pursue the division of labor between physicians and pharmacists but also to realize pharmacists' role as patient-centered family pharmacists, who integrate and review prescriptions issued by physicians, dispense independently, prevent patients from duplicated medication or drug interactions, and provide medication consultation.

To ensure pharmacists' right to dispense independently, most countries[4] that have implemented a medicine and pharmacy separation system restrict physicians with prescription rights from operating pharmacies. It is hoped that by structurally excluding physician's intervention, pharmacists could have independent space to practice.

One of the main arguments of the pharmacists to strive for in the independent pharmaceutical service is to follow the practices of advanced Western countries. But this argument over-simplifies the purpose of this important policy. What is the problem with not separating medicine and pharmacy? Is the separation a suitable strategy to tackle these problems? Will new problems produce the strategy? All of these questions have to be assessed objectively so that the medical profession and the pharmaceutical personnel will not fall into a dispute caused by personal feelings. Because of the space limitation, this article only discusses from the viewpoint of the NHI.

---

[4] Countries such as Germany, France, Italy, Belgium, the Netherlands, Denmark, Norway, Finland, Spain, and Sweden enforce the implementation of the separating medicine and pharmacy through legislation. Separation of medicine and pharmacy is not mandatory in countries such as Switzerland, Poland, the Czech Republic, the Philippines, Australia, and New Zealand but actually implemented.

The Effectiveness of Separating Medicine and Pharmacy

The result of separating medicine and pharmacy since the implementation of Article 102 of the Pharmaceutical Affairs Act can be observed from the following data:

1. Drug fee:

    Two of the reasons[5] for separating medicine and pharmacy are to avoid drug abuse and reduce drug fees. However, NHI outpatient drug fees increased annually between 2010 and 2017 and the average drug fee per claim also showed a general increase[6], which did not support the assumption empirically.

2. Drug fee claimed by the pharmacies:

    Among the NHI drug fees mentioned above, physician-released prescriptions claimed by the contracted pharmacies also increased annually from 2010 to 2017[7]. Although most hospitals had hired their own pharmacists, the number of prescriptions released from the hospitals and its proportion in the total amount of drug fees claimed by the pharmacies both increased from 2010 to 2017[8]. As most of the medical flow of hospital outpatient visits involves filling prescriptions at the in-hospital pharmacy after making a payment, it can be assumed that the possibility of patients voluntarily requesting the release of prescriptions increases and their autonomy is relatively improved. The number of prescriptions released

---

[5] The purposes for the separation of medicine and pharmacy are roughly as follows: (1) Safeguard people's right to know about the drugs they take. (2) Physician and pharmacist both perform their duties and cooperate together. (3) It is convenient for patients to fill prescriptions. (4) Integrates drugs to avoid drug abuse and reducing drug fees. (5) Follow the advanced countries and take back the dispensing right for pharmacists. (6) Reduce the workload of physicians. The reasons for not supporting the separation of medicine and pharmacy are roughly as follows: (1) It is inconvenient to fill prescriptions at a pharmacy after seeing the doctor. (2) The medical and pharmaceutical communities will compete with each other for their interests. (3) Physicians cannot control the quality and efficacy of medications after prescribing a prescription. (4) The society has insufficient awareness of the separation of medicine and pharmacy. (5) People may directly buy drugs at the pharmacy when they have the same symptoms next time, which increases the risk.

[6] There are many reasons for the increase in the NHI drug fees, such as expenses of severe and rare diseases and the introduction of high-priced new drugs. It may not be that the separation of medicine and pharmacy has not played a role. It can only say that the specific effects of the separation of medicine and pharmacy in reducing drug fees cannot be seen from the data.

[7] The number of drug fees claimed by the NHI contracted pharmacies from 2010 to 2017 were 68.153 million, 74.025 million, 76.007 million, 79.059 million, 82.552 million, 83.911 million, 88.850 million, and 91.499 million respectively. The number of RVU applications is 20.69 billion, 23.72 billion, 24.16 billion, 27.54 billion, 29.83 billion, 30.89 billion, 33.19 billion, and 35.34 billion.

[8] The number of pharmacies' drug fee claims whose prescriptions came from hospitals from 2010 to 2017 were 8.059 million, 9.41 million, 10.79 million, 12.552 million, 13.751 million, 15.126 million, 16.599 million, and 17.934 million. The proportion of drug fee claims whose prescriptions were released from hospitals in total pharmacy drug fee claims has gradually increased from 12% to about 20% year by year.

by Western medical clinics has also grown year by year[9], which is in line with the assumption mentioned above.

3. Number of the NHI-contracted pharmacies:

In 2004, there were only 3898 NHI-contracted pharmacies, and the number grew annually to 5037 in 2011 and 6203 in 2017. The increase in hospital-released prescriptions expanded the drug-dispensing market for contracted pharmacies, and the number of the contracted pharmacies increased subsequently.

Available data demonstrate that although the separation of medicine and pharmacy does not have the function of regulating overall drug fees, the number of prescriptions that hospitals issue increases in contracted pharmacies. It shows that over the past 20 years, the policy has gradually affected the habits of patients, so that they are now willing to have prescriptions filled in community pharmacies.

Ownership of Dispensing Rights from a Legal Perspective

Regarding whether the physician or the pharmacist is more eligible to the dispense drugs, both parties have their own legal right according to the current law:

1. Physicians:

   A. Article 66 of the Medical Care Act: when dispensing medications to patients, a hospital or clinic shall clearly indicate the patient's name, sex, dosage, quantity, method of administration, actions or indications, warnings or side effects of the medication, the name and location of the medical institution, the name of the dispenser and the date of dispensation on the container or package.

   B. Article 13 of the Physicians Act: when issuing prescriptions, physicians shall clearly state the following on the signed or sealed prescription slip: physician's full name, patient name, age, name of medication, dosage, amount, use and year, month and day on which the prescription was issued.

   C. Article 14 of the Physicians Act: when delivering medicines to patients, physicians have the same obligation to include necessary information such as states in Article 66 of the Medical Care Act.

2. Pharmacists:

   A. Article 37 of the Pharmaceutical Affairs Act: dispensation of drugs shall not be performed unless it follows established operational procedures; the operational guidelines shall be established by the central competent health

---

[9] The number of prescriptions released by Western primary clinics and claimed by pharmacies from 2010 to 2017 were 56.386 million, 60.727 million, 61.093 million, 62.145 million, 63.985 million, 63.846 million, 67.256 million, and 68.237 million. The proportion of drug fee claims whose prescriptions were released by Western primary clinics in total pharmacy drug fee claims has decreased from 80% to about 75% year by year.

authority. (Item 1) The aforesaid dispensation of drugs shall be performed by a pharmacist. ... (Item 2) Article 102: any physician having dispensation facilities as specified in this Act may, for the purpose of medical treatment, dispense drugs by himself/herself based on his/her own prescriptions (Item 1). After 2 years of the implementation of the National Health Insurance, the provision of the preceding Paragraph shall be enforceable only in remote areas, where practicing pharmaceutical personnel are not available as announced by the central or municipal competent health authorities or in the case of urgent need of medical treatment services (Item 2).

B. Article 50 of the Pharmaceutical Affairs Act Enforcement Rules: "Urgent need of medical treatment services," as used in Article 102, Paragraph 2 of the Act, means circumstances in which a physician at a medical care institution, owing to an urgent need for medical care measures, must immediately use a drug.

C. Articles 12, 15 to 20, and 20–21 of the Pharmacists Act specify the pharmacist's obligations to dispense medications, precautions, regulations to comply with when dispensing medication, and their right to administer dispensation business, etc.

D. Good dispensing practice specifies the personnel (pharmacists, assistant pharmacists), procedures and equipment required for drug dispensation.

Judging from the Medical Care Act and the Physicians Act above, physicians have the right to issue prescriptions. Although none of the laws mentioned whether physicians have the right to dispense prescriptions, they have the obligation to deliver prescriptions. Actions including preparation, compounding, and confirmation of the drugs that must be completed before drug deliveries are defined as being within the scope of "dispensation"[10]. Therefore, physicians should complete a series of procedures including prescribing, preparing, compounding, and confirming drugs and delivering them to patients. Moreover, the scope of the physician's dispensation is limited to prescriptions prescribed by himself or herself. That means, even with statutory equipment, physicians are not allowed to dispense drugs for other physicians.

Of course, objections have been voiced that the Physicians Act and the Medical Care Act only regulate the delivery of drugs by physicians, which is only one part of the dispensation; therefore, physicians are not allowed to conduct other parts of the dispensation[11]. The pharmaceutical professionals argue that, in accordance with Article 102, Item 2 of the Pharmaceutical Affairs Act (announced on 5 February 1993), 2 years after the implementation of the NHI, physicians have no right to

---

[10] According to Article 3 of Good Dispensing Practices, Dispensation shall mean the activities performed by any pharmacist or assisting pharmacist that involve prescription verification, prescription registration, assessment of the appropriateness of drug administration, preparation or compounding of any drug, reverification, confirmation of drug delivery to any recipient, and instructions for drug administration during the period between the time when the pharmacy practitioner receives any prescription to the time when the patient acquires the drug.

[11] Take the Supreme Administrative Court's Judgment No. 971 in 2005 as an example.

dispensation, except for in remote areas or medical emergencies. This is the principle that the later law has priority over the earlier law [1]. However, Article 14 of the Physicians Act stated in 1967 that physicians should properly label the medication when they deliver the drugs and the revision of the Article in 2002 did not delete this regulation. Instead, to protect the patient's right to know, the scope of information that physicians should label was expanded. The same principle was applied in the amendment of Article 66 of the Medical Care Act in 2004, and the abovementioned regulation was added. If the later law has priority over the earlier law, it is hard to recognize the Pharmaceutical Affairs Act as the later one. In addition, comparing Article 102 of the Pharmaceutical Affairs Act with the relevant regulation in the Physicians Act and the Medical Care Act, it is difficult to conclude that Article 102 of the Pharmaceutical Affairs Law is a special law that should be applied first. There are indeed unresolved conflicts regarding the ownership of the dispensation rights in the provisions of the above regulations.

The judicial community also has different opinions on whether physicians can dispense the prescription in general after the implementation of Article 102 of the Pharmacists Act. There is a case involving a clinic that did not hire pharmaceutical personnel, and the drugs were delivered by the physician in charge. The health bureau of the competent authority fined the physician for violation of the provisions of the Pharmaceutical Affairs Act. The Taichung High Administrative Court ruled that the plaintiff's physician won the case. There are three reasons:

1. Whether the physician delivers the drugs belongs to the scope of dispensation. The so-called dispensation is only defined in Article 2 of "Good Dispensing Practice" based on the Pharmaceutical Affairs Act Enforcement Rules[12] at the time of the action, not authorized by law. The definition of dispensation in Article 37 of the Pharmaceutical Affairs Act, which is only an administrative rule issued by administrative agencies in order to enforce the rules, violates the principle of clarity of authorization.
2. Article 14 of the Physicians Act, an act that was amended and announced later, is still part of the physician's obligation to deliver drugs to patients. Therefore, delivering drugs to patients by physicians is permitted by the law. The competent authority's restriction on physicians' right to dispense in urgent situations only in Article 14 of the Physicians Act is a limited interpretation. However, Article 14 and all the provisions of the Physicians Act are difficult to serve as the basis of the limited interpretation.
3. The physician's dispensation is not equivalent to dispensation made by the medical layman. Article 37, Item 2 of the Pharmaceutical Affairs Act stipulates that the dispensation of drugs should be carried out by pharmacists. However, the Act is also stipulated in Item 1, Article 102 that physicians may dispense drugs, subject to the restrictions specified in Item 2. This could not be seen in the same way

---

[12] Article 20 of the Pharmaceutical Affairs Act Enforcement Rules was deleted on 16 February 2005, and Article 37 of the Pharmaceutical Affairs Act clearly authorized the establishment of Good Dispensing Practice, but both have the same definition of dispensation.

as the possible risk and harm to patient's health caused by drugs dispensed by the medical layman. It is questionable whether the intention of the legislation is betrayed when the competent authority recognizes both of the situations violated in Article 37, Item 2 of the Pharmaceutical Affairs Act.

After the appeal of this case, the competent authority won a reversal. The Supreme Administrative Court's Judgment No. 971 in 2005 held that:

1. Both physicians and pharmacists have professional licenses, and each has its own scope of practice. The process of a physician treating patients starts from diagnosis and ends in providing medication. The dispensing of medication, which involves the pharmacist's expertise, includes the preparation and the delivery of drugs. However, the preparation and delivery of drugs according to the needs of patients are necessary for medical behaviors and are also covered by the physician's profession. Therefore, it is not unreasonable for physicians to take care of it. Based on above reasons, physicians have the right to dispense drugs when treating patients. However, after the amendment of the Pharmaceutical Affairs Act in 1993, physicians' right to dispense drugs was restricted to remote areas or under an medical emergency with the purpose of treating patients.
2. Dispensation is a professional term for pharmaceutical affairs. As the definition of dispensation is not clearly documented by law at the time of the action and does not specifically define the scope of its concept, it can be determined by the profession of pharmaceutical affairs without authorization.
3. According to Article 102 of the Pharmaceutical Affairs Act, in remote areas and medical emergencies, physicians can dispense drugs, including delivery drugs. In addition, in accordance with Article 14 of the Physicians Act, a physician is eligible to deliver drugs by hiring pharmacists in-house to dispense drugs. The delivery of drugs is part of the dispensing procedure, and the drugs delivered by physicians must be dispensed by the pharmacist. This does not mean that the physicians have the right to dispense drugs in accordance with Article 14 of the Physicians Act; otherwise, it will impact the separation of medicine and pharmacy.

After the Supreme Administrative Court made the above judgment, more judgments such as the Miaoli District Court's Judgment No. 28 in 2014 and the Taipei District Court's Judgment No. 195 in 2017 reflected the same opinions as those of the Supreme Administrative Court.

Although the Supreme Administrative Court agrees that Article 102 of the Pharmaceutical Affairs Act restricts the physician's right to dispense, it also pointed out that "according to the needs of patients, the preparation and delivery of drugs are necessary for medical behaviors, and they are also covered by the physician's profession. It is not unreasonable for the physician to take care of it." Therefore, it is not quite reasonable for the competent authority to equate "physician's dispensation" with "layman's dispensation."

The Person in Charge of Medical Services in the National Health Insurance System

Physicians and pharmacists are professional and technical personnel, and they must pass exams in order to practice. The state requests that certain jobs must be performed by individuals with qualifications because of the content and nature of the work involving important public welfare and a high level of proficiency; thus, the corresponding performer must possess professional knowledge and experience. At the same time, in order to protect the public welfare and the rights and interests of the professional personnel, the state will also impose penalties on those without qualification and execute the scope of practice.

The right to dispense was regarded as the core practice of pharmacists at the beginning of the legislation of the Pharmacists Act. Judging those who have pharmaceutical expertise from their professional competence and scope of professional practice, pharmacists are most qualified and authorized to determine the best medication and usage for patients and take responsibility. Those who advocate for the separation of medicine and pharmacy assert that pharmacists can confirm and supervise the prescriptions from physicians; however, this conflict is within the scope of practice and responsibilities of physicians.

The healthcare service in our country is characterized by the strong bond between patients and physicians, and patients are highly dependent on physicians. Therefore, there is no doubt that physicians bear the ultimate and almost full responsibility for the treatment of patients. Once the health outcome is not satisfactory, the physicians are always the subject of prosecution[13]. When managing contracted medical institutions, the NHIA also holds medical personnel who are in charge of the institution accountable. Exceptions occur when there are medical personnel who are responsible for specific violations; then, the punishment will be imposed simultaneously. Except for the contracted pharmacies, the person in charge of the contracted medical institution is always a physician.

After diagnosing and issuing a prescription, the physician still has to track and adjust the prescription according to the effect of treatment and medication. If the prescription has been integrated, replaced, increased, or decreased by pharmacists, obstacles and blind spots will inevitably arise. When the physician follows up on the condition of the disease and adjusts treatment methods accordingly, the risk of medical disputes and legal liabilities thereby increases. Therefore, the NHIA established the NHI MediCloud System to share pharmacists' responsibility of integrating

---

[13] According to the medical personnel involved in the statistics of medical disputes in E-Da Hospital from 2001 to 2003, Western physicians accounted for 82%, nursing staff accounted for 6%, dentists accounted for 2%, traditional Chinese medicine physicians accounted for 2%, pharmacists accounted for 4%, examiners 1.8%, and others 2.2%. Physicians account for the absolute majority of the subjects to prosecution from patients and their families. In addition, refer to the "Medical Appraisal Medical Litigation," the Joint Commission of Taiwan, December 2013, even if the case involved disputes the appropriateness of medication, physicians and hospitals were mostly the subjects of prosecution.

medicines and avoiding duplication by checking patient's medication records from different medical facilities in the past few months. The system automatically alters the physicians if the drugs they are going to prescribe duplicate or interact with the patient's current medicine to effectively reduce the probability of such problems.

Article 17 of the Pharmaceutical Affairs Act stipulates that the pharmacist should dispense the drugs according to the prescription. If the medicine is not available or is lacking, the pharmacist should inform the physician who prescribed the medicine regarding a replacement instead of omitting or substituting medicines arbitrarily. The clause echoes the physician's right to prescribe and the fact that the physician is responsible for the medical process. If the pharmacist has to follow the physician's prescription completely, according to the above provisions, the pharmacist can only discuss and give opinions to the physician at most. The physician still has the right to decide whether to change the prescription or not. Then, in a system in which drug prescribing and dispensing are separate, the "review, supervision, check and balance" function of a pharmacist when they are "evaluating the physician's diagnosis, verifying whether duplication exists, interaction, individual contraindications, potential side effects, and rationality of medications, and others" is very limited. Besides the pharmacists, other medical personnel also have to "follow the physician's orders" when providing medical services at all times, so there is limited room for independent business execution.

Besides physicians and pharmacists, other professionals have an overlapping scope of practice. For example, bookkeepers and accountants have their own scope of practice, but both can execute tax business[14].

One of the purposes of separating medicine and pharmacy is to promote the pharmacists' independent practice and to serve patients better. However, under the current conditions, physicians are the leaders of planning medical services and almost the only people who are responsible. Therefore, the failure to achieve the goal of separating medicine and pharmacy in one step is a reality that requires understanding.

The Strategy to Promote Separation of Medicine and Pharmacy—Discussion and Conclusions

Before the implementation of the separation of medicine and pharmacy, these two parts of the services were intertwined in the Western medical healthcare process in Taiwan [3]. The scope of practice of physicians includes diagnosis, treatment, prescriptions, and dispensation, covering most of the medical services. In addition, medical economic research also pointed out that medical service is obviously characterized by monopolistic competition and information asymmetry, leading to

---

[14] Refer to Article 13 of the Certified Public Bookkeepers Act and Article 39 of the Certified Public Accountant Act.

patients' limited ability in seeking alternative services. Consequently, the bonding between patients and physicians continuously strengthens throughout the medical process, and the relationship between patients, nurses, pharmacists, medical technologists, and other medical personnel remains relatively weak. If the physicians do not actively release the prescriptions, patients usually will not request this; most people's decision-making process for choosing pharmacies is directed by the physician's instructions [2]. This is also the reason why the front-door pharmacies were so popular when the policy was just implemented.

Therefore, considering the historical factors, research results, and empirical situation of medicine and pharmacy development, society highly relies on physicians in the whole medical process, and it is not easy to change the habits of the whole of society simply by separating medicine and pharmacy. The pharmaceutical professionals actively advocate the single-track separation of medicine and pharmacy and appeal to impose legal enforcement. Embedding important policy into law is certainly one of the more feasible methods. However, concerning the habituation of society, and the separation of medicine and pharmacy, specific arguments coupled with positive policy incentives can gradually cultivate a social environment conducive to the implementation of the policy. The proliferation of front-door pharmacies that has been attributed to the increasing RVUs of prescription releases highlights that such results may be difficult to achieve with regulations alone. Only legal systems constructed under a mature social environment, which can promote policies, act as a stitch in time saves nine.

Sociologists point out that in addition to the economic benefits it brings, workload division also meets the needs of society. Besides establishing the relationship between different professions, we also have to invigorate individual professions and the "spontaneous division of labor" can form [2] only in this way. The same goes for the separation of medicine and pharmacy. The professionals should demonstrate their specialization by increasing drug safety and additional new values to the publics. When the public recognize the value of independent pharmaceutical service, they would become active collaborators rather than passive recipients and transform the separation of medicine and pharmacy into a social demand. Demand will guide services, and differentiated medical services will follow the trend.

There is no doubt that the NHI shapes the medical environment in Taiwan. To promote the established policy of separating medicine and pharmacy, the NHI will fully utilize the system and promote the core values of pharmacists to accelerate transformation of healthcare-seeking behavior. Before the ideal single-track division is realized, pharmacists can still seize the chance to show their expertise in the current medical environment dominated by physicians. As our society ages, the demand for home and community medical care is rising and people need not only family physicians but also family pharmacists who may be closer to their lives. In addition to performing core responsibilities such as guaranteeing drug safety, pharmacists could also transform pharmacies into important bases of the care system that exert multifaceted functions, creating more value and contributions.

Patient-Centered Integrated Care Plans[15]

Taiwan officially became an "aged society" when the proportion of the population aged 65 and above reached 14% of the total population in March 2018. In addition, we have only 8 years left to reach the "super-aged society" (the population aged 65 and above makes up more than 20% of the total population), which further reflects the severity of ageing in our country. The NHIA has planned a number of policies in recent years to prepare for the medical needs of the super-aged society that Taiwan will face in the future. The elderly often take multiple medications, have comorbidities, and exhibit characteristics of "geriatric syndrome" such as physical and mental deterioration and disability. Therefore, the NHIA proactively implements various integrated medical service plans to construct a patient-centered healthcare system.

National Health Insurance Big Data Reflect the Ageing Population

With an ageing population, technology advancement, and medical progress, the average life expectancy of Taiwanese people increases continuously, and the most prevalent type of disease has gradually changed from acute disease caused by bacterial and virus infection to a chronic disease caused by lifestyle. However, the treatment of chronic disease is different from that of acute disease whereas most of the time the treatments only stabilized the condition rather than curing the disease. Therefore, as the number of patients with chronic diseases increases, their follow-up medical care poses challenges to the NHI.

According to the analysis of the NHI big data, the number of patients with chronic diseases and medical expenses in Taiwan has been on the rise. In 2017, medical expenses for chronic diseases have reached New Taiwan dollars (NTD) 231.8 billion, accounting for about 30% of the total, and an increase of 23% from 2013 (Fig. 4.1). The number of chronic disease patients in 2017 has exceeded 6 million, which equates to a quarter of the total population and represents a 13% increase from 2013.

In addition, the outpatient medical expenses per person for the 65-and-older population reveals that the expenditure for chronic disease drugs is around NTD 33 billion, and the medical expenses are more than NTD 60 billion, both are much higher than the expenses for those aged between 19 and 64 years old (NTD 9.3 billion and NTD 16.5 billion respectively), the working age population. In view of this, as the working age population gradually becomes the elderly in the future, the medical expenditures of the NHI will be more substantial.

---

[15] 201903 Public Governance Quarterly.

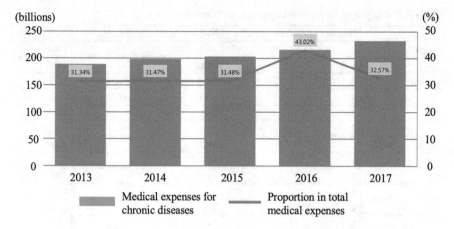

Fig. 4.1 Medical expenses for chronic diseases and their proportion in total medical expenses. (Source: National Health Insurance Administration)

Statistics from the NHIA show that the number of chronic disease patients is 6.29 million in 2017, among them, 3.86 million are people aged 65 and above, accounting for about 60%. When we further analyze the data by the number of chronic diseases they have, there are 2.13 million people suffering from one kind of chronic disease, accounting for about 34%, and the remaining 66% suffer from more than two kinds of chronic diseases. In addition, nearly 60% of people who are aged 65 years or older have multiple chronic diseases (Table 4.1). This shows that the number of people suffering from chronic diseases in the country is increasing year by year, and patients with chronic disease who visit doctors in different hospitals or departments are likely to have duplicate prescriptions. These duplicate prescriptions do not just waste medical resources. Medications exceeding their safe dosages or interacting with medications prescribed by other physicians pose risks to patient health.

The Family Doctor Integrated Care Program

Because of the abundance of medical resources in the domestic metropolitan area and the low co-payment required in the NHI system, many people visit doctors but still fail to obtain a proper diagnosis and treatment. Therefore, The NHIA implemented the "Family Doctor Integrated Care Program" in 2003 to encourage at least five clinics in the same area to form a "community healthcare group" with partner hospitals. It is hoped that through the implementation of the Family Doctor Integrated Care Program, people will develop correct healthcare-seeking behavior. The public will receive primary care provided by primary clinics on a regular basis and get referred to the hospital for medical treatment when further diagnosis and

Table 4.1 Analysis of the number of patients with chronic diseases in 2017

	Number of chronic diseases	Number of people (thousands)	Percentage
Total		6289	100%
	1	2127	34%
	2	2013	32%
	3	1200	19%
	4	578	9%
	5	371	6%
Aged under 65		2429	100%
	1	561	23%
	2	740	30%
	3	564	23%
	4	323	13%
	5	242	10%
Aged over 65		3859	100%
	1	1566	41%
	2	1273	33%
	3	636	16%
	4	255	7%
	5	129	3%

Notes:
1. The data are from the second-generation warehouse of the NHIA
2. Definition of chronic disease: the main diagnosis in an outpatient is one of the 100 chronic diseases announced by the NHIA, the same person has seen the doctor more than twice, and there are more than 60 annual dosing days

treatment is necessary, integrating medical resources in hospitals and primary clinics.

Under the "Family Doctor Integrated Care Program," primary clinics cooperate with contracted hospitals to provide more comprehensive health care, including the 24-h consultation hotline services for members of this plan. The aim is to reduce emergency room and unnecessary visits by providing appropriate health education and value-added services. The NHIA also established a comprehensive referral mechanism to improve the continuity and coordination of patient care by implementing the two-way referral and collaborative care. We evaluate the service provision, healthcare quality, satisfaction, preventive care, and link the performance to the NHI payment system to ensure the smooth operation of the plan.

A total of 526 community medical groups in Taiwan participated in the "Family Doctor Integrated Care Program" by the end of 2017. There were 4063 primary clinics participating, an increase of 1006 from 3057 in 2016. Approximately 2.5 million people received health care in this plan in 2015, and the number increased to 4.1 million in 2017, showing a 1.6-fold increase in 3 years. Medical expenses of 2015 and 2017 were NTD 1.2 billion and 2 billion respectively, representing a 1.7-fold increase during this period (Table 4.2).

Table 4.2 Number of cases and medical utilization of the "Family Doctor Integrated Care Program" from 2015 to 2017

Item	Year		
	2015	2016	2017
Total RVUs (million NTD)	1180	1180	2030
Number of clinics	3035	3057	4063
Number of physicians	3709	3789	5182
Number of community medical groups	426	414	526
Number of cases (thousands)	2485	2604	4134

Source: NHIA
RVU relative value unit, *NTD* New Taiwan dollar

Providing a New Model of Integration and Interdisciplinary Services

The NHIA provides integrated medical services for patients with multiple chronic diseases, hoping that the comprehensive, coordinated, and continuous medical care helps to improve safety and avoid duplication as well as improper medication and treatment. In addition, the NHIA offers additional integrated medical services in different levels of medical institutions to cater to the healthcare-seeking behavior of the public. If patients are accustomed to visiting hospitals, they can participate in the "Patient-Centered Integrated Outpatient Care Program in Hospitals"; if patients are used to seeking treatment in the clinics, they can join the "Family Doctor Integrated Care Program." Patients with impaired mobility for whom it is not convenient to obtain medical treatment in hospitals or clinics can participate in the "Integrated Home Health Care Program."

Since 2009, the NHIA has implemented the "Patient-Centered Integrated Outpatient Care Program in Hospitals" to foster proper integration of various specialties in the hospital and encourage hospitals not only to think about treatment strategies from the scope of a single medical department, but to provide integrated outpatient care services. The hospitals integrate medical teams by providing medical services from multiple specialized physicians. Each consultation accounts for at least 3 h, or by providing a one-stop consultation service for patients with dementia, major injuries or rare diseases, multiple chronic conditions of the elderly, chronic conditions (such as high blood pressure, high blood lipids, and high blood glucose), and other diseases. In addition to the general consultation fee for each visit, an additional outpatient integration fee will be awarded. As for an integrated outpatient clinic that is provided by multidisciplinary doctors, an additional fee will be awarded; for patients with dementia, 300–500 RVUs are paid for family consultation. Through economic incentives, The NHIA provides integrated care service to patients with multiple chronic conditions, hoping to improve the quality of care, so that the public can feel more at ease while seeing a doctor when the quality of healthcare is guaranteed.

Table 4.3 Number of cases and medical utilization of the "Patient-Centered Integrated Outpatient Care Program in Hospitals" from 2015 to 2017

	Year		
Item	2015	2016	2017
Total RVUs (million NTD)	112.9	228.0	228.0
Number of hospitals	188	188	189
Number of cases	359,260	553,742	522,330

Source: NHIA

RVU relative value units, *NTD* New Taiwan dollars

According to the statistics, 189 hospitals participated in the "Patient-Centered Integrated Outpatient Care Program in Hospitals" in 2017. The number of cases increased from 360,000 to 520,000 from 2015 to 2017, and the number has increased by 1.4 times in 3 years. Medical expenses increased from about NTD 110 million in 2015 to about NTD 230 million in 2017, and the cost has doubled (Table 4.3).

Incorporating the Labor Power of Home Care into Integrated Care

To further serve patients with impaired mobility, the NHIA has been seeking funding to promote the "Integrated Home Health Care Program" since 2016. For elderly and disabled persons with impaired mobility, the care team in community evaluates and integrates care resources before long-term care staff provide life care services, and medical personnel can provide home medical care for them. The service extends to home hospice and palliative care as the patients' conditions shift, to care for them at the end of life in a patient-centered manner.

The "Integrated Home Health Care Program" comprises general home care, home respiratory care, home hospice care, and the home medical care plan that was trialed in 2015. Through the cooperation of care teams and the case management mechanism, the NHIA provides patients with complete medical services. The continuity of home medical care is therefore enhanced when patients do not have to change the care team when their health conditions change.

A total of 195 teams and 2024 hospitals participated in 2017, covering all 50 medical sub-regions, and more than 90% were primary clinics and home care, which can provide care nearby. The cumulative number of participants in 2017 was 32,759. Among them, 85.4% are over 65 years old, and this is 4.3 times higher than the 7675 people receiving service between March and December in 2016. Medical expenses have increased by seven times, from NTD 60 million in 2016 to NTD 470 million in 2017 (Table 4.4).

Starting from 2019, the "Integrated Home Health Care Program" has expanded its scope and started to include services provided by dentists, Chinese medicine physicians, and pharmacists. At the same time, the responsibility of home care

Table 4.4 Number of cases and medical utilization of the "Integrated Home Health Care Program" from 2016 to 2017

Item	Year	
	2016	2017
Total RVUs (million NTD)	66.0	469.5
Number of teams	106	195
Number of institutions	550	2024
Cumulative number of cases	7645	32,759

Source: NHIA
RVU relative value unit, *NTD* New Taiwan dollars

doctors has been further emphasized. The home care doctor is responsible for evaluating a patient's overall needs for home care, and requesting services provided by other medical personnel, such as dentists, Chinese medicine physicians, nurses, and respiratory therapists, when necessary. Patients are required to cooperate with home care doctors in medication reconciliation and comprehensive home care. If the patient cannot cooperate with the doctor, he or she shall return to receive medicine during outpatient sessions, so that the limited number of home care service providers can take care of physically impaired patients with actual needs.

Promoting the Vertical Integration of Hospitals and Clinics

The implementation of the "Family Doctor Integrated Care Program," the "Patient-Centered Integrated Outpatient Care Program in Hospitals," the "Integrated Home Health Care Program," and various programs of the NHI is aimed at improving medical accessibility and quality to construct a patient-centered medical care system, by providing patients with safe, appropriate, and continuous integrated medical services according to their needs, and to reduce the waste of medical resources.

The tiered medical care system and two-way referral, which NHIA has proactively promoted since 2017, have received enthusiastic responses from the majority of medical centers and regional hospitals. They have come forward to take the leading role by forming alliances with community hospitals and clinics actively in their areas. As of mid-November 2018, there was a total of 78 "vertical integration" strategic alliance groups of institutes in Taiwan. The NHIA encourages people to seek medical care from their trusted family doctors nearby when they are not feeling well. As the primary clinics have medical centers as their medical backup, referrals can be arranged through the "Electronic Referral Platform" established by the NHIA when necessary. The division of workload and cooperation between clinics and hospitals not only provides continuous care for patients, but also reduces their cost and time spent traveling to and waiting in big hospitals.

Healthcare Digital Transformation Brings Win–Win–Win for Physicians, Patients, and National Health Insurance

With limited NHI resources, the NHIA and the medical profession must reach a consensus on how to design incentives that support the integrated care services and reward systems that pay according to the service quality. Some representatives of the medical profession complained that under the current division of medical specialties, it is difficult to provide integrated care services from physicians with different expertise. Some hospitals provide integrated care services, whereas in fact they only integrate the medical information, so patients still have to visit multiple departments. Some patients hope to maintain the freedom of choosing their medical providers. Because of the above-mentioned factors, the medical care system is still facing challenges in fragmentation.

In recent years, the NHIA has been actively integrating various sorts of medical information, such as the establishment of the "NHI PharmaCloud System" in 2016 to ensure the safety of patients' medications and avoid duplicate medications. It was upgraded to the "NHI MediCloud System" in 2017, providing additional medical information including examination and test records and results. The NHIA established the "Medical Image Sharing and Access" mechanism in 2018 to provide clinicians with real-time cross-hospital access to patients' digital medical images, and has further set up an online real-time reminder, so that the clinician can immediately review the medication and examination (test) patients received in the last 3–6 months before ordering new ones. If every physician can query the NHI MediCloud System in the clinic thoroughly to avoid duplicate examinations and medications, unnecessary medical expenses can be reduced, and patient safety can also be guaranteed.

In recent years, the NHIA has carried out various medical and expenditure reforms to distribute the medical and NHI resources more effectively, and reduced medical waste by managing its source, hoping to avoid the impact on income of medical staff caused by the RVU fluctuation attributed to the global payment system (Fig. 4.2). In addition, the NHIA improved the mobile phone authentication function of "My Health Bank" in 2018 to support people's self-health management. The public can download the National Health Insurance Mobile Easy Access mobile application (NHI Express App) to check personal insurance premium payment and medical records, health examinations, preventive health care, and other related information easily. By the end of 2021, the number of downloads had exceeded 7 million. We hope to create a win–win–win situation for physicians, patients, and the NHI so as to meet the challenges of the super-aged society.

Connection to Long-Term Care After Hospital Discharge

To provide comprehensive and continuous care after hospital discharge, the NHIA continues to support contracted hospitals in improving the quality of the discharge planning service. We look forward to providing high-quality discharge planning

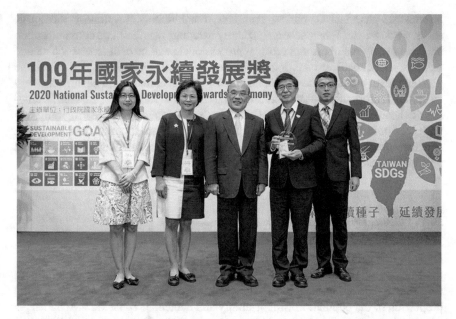

Fig. 4.2 The NHIA won the 2020 National Sustainability Award with the theme of "Digitalized Health Network—the NHI MediCloud"

through cross-organization cooperation, so that inpatients who have needs for long-term care can receive necessary services in a timely manner.

Covering the Discharge Planning and Follow-Up Management Fee Through National Health Insurance

The NHIA provides patients with needs assessment, health education, and interprofessional communication during their hospitalization. The services also include coordination of information as well as referral arrangement for subsequent medical follow-ups, long-term care and social resources to reduce the possibility of emergency revisit and readmission shortly after their discharge. The "Discharge Planning and Follow-up Management Fee" was added to the NHI fee schedule in April 2016, so that 1500 RVUs are paid per person per time. The NHIA stipulated the subject eligibility and established the specifications and procedures in June 2017 as operational guides that hospitals could follow and properly connect hospital discharge with follow-up care services.

Most hospitals provide discharge planning by their in-house discharge planning team. The case managers customize discharge plans for specific inpatients and conduct at least one interprofessional communication meeting depending on the patients' condition. Participants of the discharge planning team may include physicians, pharmacists, nurses, dietitians, rehabilitators, respiratory therapists, social workers, etc. When necessary, family meetings that facilitate communication between family members and medical professionals will be held to assess patients' post-discharge medical care, long-term care, or other social need. The discharge planning team provides the patient and their family members with health education and related information, as well as arranging referral to follow-up care such as community healthcare groups in the NHI Family Doctor Integrated Care Program, various types of home care, the Integrated Home Health Care Program, and long-term care institutions. The service also includes more than one telephone follow-up and telephone consultation within 2 weeks after discharge.

Implementation of Long-Term Care 2.0

Owing to the aging population in Taiwan and the diversified needs for care services, the Ministry of Health and Welfare has established a community-based long-term care service system in response to the need for long-term care for the increasing proportion of the population with disability and dementia. To tackle the challenges of long-term care in our aging society, the "National Ten-Year Long-Term Care Plan 2.0" (referred to as Long-Term Care 2.0) was approved by Executive Yuan in December 2016 and put into effect in January 2017.

In addition to promotion of the Comprehensive Community Care and development of innovative services, the Long-Term Care 2.0 also focuses on the establishment of a community-based healthcare team, and connection to other services such as discharge planning and home medical service.

Connection Between National Health Insurance Discharge Planning and Long-Term Care 2.0

The goal of the "Discharge Planning and Long-Term Care 2.0 Connection Friendly Hospital Reward Program" and the "2020 Discharge Planning Connect to Long-Term Care Plan" is to encourage hospitals to complete a long-term care needs assessment, and referral arrangement to the long-term care facilities before patients leave the hospitals, so that the long-term care services can kick in within 7 days after discharge to avoid care fragmentation. By doing so, we hope to reduce the long waiting time before the initiation of long-term care service caused by the traditional needs assessment process (Fig. 4.3).

From April 2017 to December 2020, there were a total of 508,534 claim cases from 361,708 patients regarding the "Discharge Planning and Follow-up Management Fee." Among them, 139,034 claim cases were eligible for the Long-Term Care 2.0 and assessed for their Long-Term Care 2.0 needs before or after being discharged from the hospital. Among them, 94,113 cases subsequently

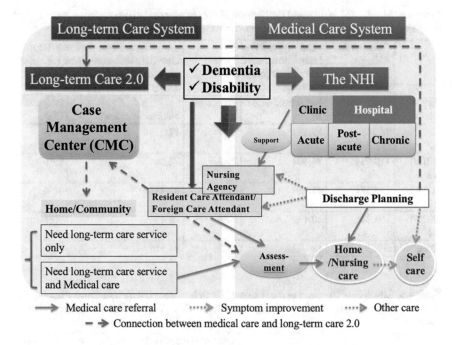

Fig. 4.3 Connection process between medical care and Long-Term Care 2.0

received the Long-Term Care 2.0 services, accounting for 68% of the total number assessed. The rate of subsequent transfers to long-term care services is increasing year by year (Table 4.5).

To understand if cases are connected to Long-Term Care 2.0 seamlessly, we conducted a subset analysis for 69,336 cases who received a needs assessment prior to discharge. Among them, 28,447 cases received the Long-Term Care 2.0 service within 7 days after discharge, accounting for 41% of the recipients of the Long-Term Care 2.0 needs assessment during their hospital stay and the proportion of this item is showing an increasing trend (Table 4.6).

Tiered Medical Care System

In Taiwan, the comprehensive coverage provided by NHI allows residents to gain easy access to medical treatment, and can freely choose the institution for medical treatment. Therefore, people tend to swarm to big hospitals regardless of whether they have serious or mild illnesses. The overcrowded situation in big hospitals causes extreme waiting times for patients with acute, severe, and difficult diseases with immediate needs for specialized care. On the other hand, it is difficult for small community hospitals to sustain themselves because of the small number of patients they serve. These two extremes have caused inefficiency in the overall medical care system, and revolutionary policies are urgently needed to improve this situation.

Table 4.5 Situation of the cases of the National Health Insurance (NHI) "Discharge Planning and Follow-up Management Fee" receiving Long-Term Care 2.0 services

Statistic period	Claim of the NHI discharge planning	Case who receives the Long-Term Care 2.0 needs assessment before or after discharge		Case who receives the Long-Term Care 2.0 needs assessment before or after discharge and Long-Term Care 2.0 services after discharge	
	Number of cases A	Number of cases B	Proportion B/A	Number of cases C	Proportion C/B
2017/4-12	78,743	19,187	24%	12,026	63%
2018/1-12	119,054	34,404	29%	22,36	65%
2019/1-12	146,391	44,984	31%	31,331	70%
2020/1-12	164,346	40,459	25%	28,450	70%
Total	508,534	139,034	27%	94,113	68%

Table 4.6 Situation of the cases of the National Health Insurance (NHI) "Discharge Planning and Follow-up Management Fee" receiving Long-Term Care 2.0 services—assessment before discharge

Statistic period	Claim of the NHI discharge planning	Case who receives the Long-Term Care 2.0 needs assessment before discharge		Case who receives the Long-Term Care 2.0 needs assessment before discharge and Long-Term Care 2.0 services within 7 days after discharge		Case who receives the Long-Term Care 2.0 needs assessment before discharge and Long-Term Care 2.0 services after discharge	
	Number of cases A	Number of cases B	Proportion B/A	Number of cases C	Proportion C/B	Number of cases D	Proportion D/B
2017/4-12	78,743	3357	4%	784	23%	2031	61%
2018/1-12	119,054	13,760	12%	4066	30%	8976	65%
2019/1-12	146,391	24,727	17%	10,667	43%	17,900	72%
2020/1-12	164,346	27,492	17%	12,930	47%	20,165	73%
Total	508,534	69,336	14%	28,447	41%	49,072	71%

The goal of the tiered medical care system is to encourage the public to seek medical care in the right way by receiving healthcare from the same provider regularly. In this way, their doctors can quickly evaluate their conditions and refer patients to appropriate hospitals for further medical treatment when necessary. Of course, the change of behaviors cannot be accomplished overnight. It must be promoted over a long period and implemented with appropriate supporting measures.

Current Distribution of Hospital Levels

The number of hospitals has shown a decreasing trend in the past 5 years. For example, in 2020, there were 25 medical centers, 82 regional hospitals, and 368 district hospitals. Compared with 2016, the most significant change was that the number of district hospitals decreased by 6. However, the number of wards increased at all hospital levels. The total number of wards increased from about 130,000 to 134,000 over the 5 years (Tables 4.7 and 4.8).

In terms of medical expenses, the total medical expenses claimed by medical centers and regional hospitals are both around 200 billion RVUs each year, whereas that of district hospitals has grown gradually to approximately 100 billion RVUs, and medical expenses of district hospitals have also slightly increased from 16.7% in 2016 to 18.7% in 2020 (Table 4.9). This may be attributed to the downgrading of the two regional hospitals to district hospitals in 2019.

Table 4.7 Statistics of the number of facilities at each hospital level in the past 5 years

Year	Medical centers	Regional hospitals	District hospitals	Total
2016	26	84	374	484
2017	26	84	369	479
2018	26	84	368	478
2019	25	82	370	477
2020	25	82	368	475

Table 4.8 Statistics on the number of wards at each hospital level in the past 5 years

Year	Medical centers		Regional hospitals		District hospitals		Total
	Acute	Chronic	Acute	Chronic	Acute	Chronic	acute and chronic
2016	31,323	715	50,313	5636	31,865	10,766	130,618
2017	31,460	759	50,295	5555	32,373	10,684	131,126
2018	31,528	772	50,820	5590	33,074	10,671	132,455
2019	31,312	769	49,996	5590	34,249	10,365	132,281
2020	31,344	769	50,468	5606	35,540	10,347	134,074

Table 4.9 Statistics on the number of medical expenses claimed by each hospital level in the past 5 years

Year	Medical centers		Regional hospitals		District hospitals		Total
	RVUs (100 million)	Percentage	RVUs (100 million)	Percentage	RVUs (100 million)	Percentage	RVUs (100 million)
2016	1866	42.7%	1778	40.7%	728	16.7%	4374
2017	1997	42.8%	1893	40.5%	782	16.7%	4673
2018	2115	42.6%	1995	40.2%	855	17.2%	4965
2019	2202	42.2%	2057	39.4%	957	18.4%	5218
2020	2241	42.3%	2065	39.0%	993	18.7%	5300

RVU relative value unit

Encouraging Big Hospitals to Treat Acute, Severe, and Difficult Diseases

The hospitals are divided into three levels in the NHI: medical center, regional hospital, and district hospital. Medical centers and regional hospitals, commonly known as "big hospitals," are staffed not only by various specialists but even by subspecialists. Besides that, they have a wide range of examination and test equipment and advanced instruments. Big hospitals are able to provide high-quality medical services for inpatients and patients with acute, severe, and difficult diseases with the highly specialized human resources and equipment they possess. Therefore, the NHI, with a strong backing for big hospitals, is obligated to provide big hospitals with strong support in term of reimbursement.

Because of the difficulty of treatment for acute, severe, and difficult diseases, the big hospitals demand more security in their human resources. Therefore, the NHIA strives to utilize the limited NHI resources to not only increase the reimbursement of diagnosis, treatment, and surgery related to acute, severe, and difficult diseases continuously, but also secure the value of the RVU. Starting from 2021, the NHIA planned to first adopt a fixed RVU value to guarantee the inpatient examination fee, nursing fee, and ward fee of the intensive care ward, and then obtains a budget in the following years to gradually expand the scope of coverage.

Small Hospitals Are the Leaders of Community Medical Care

The most fundamental level of the pyramid of the tiered medical care system is the primary health care from community medical institutions. Community medical care is provided by all primary clinics and small hospitals in the community. Based on 368 million outpatient visits in 2019, about 71 million medical visits were made in big hospitals (medical centers and regional hospitals), which means that 297 million medical visits accounting for 80% of total outpatient visits, occurred in community medical institutes.

To promote the "good doctors in the community" policy, district hospitals, as the big brothers of community medical care, not only cooperate with the promotion of "Holiday Clinics in District Hospital" to share the congestion in emergency departments of big hospitals but also continuously improve the lineup of their doctors. In addition to inviting doctors from big hospitals to support outpatient clinics, the district hospitals also actively join the medical alliance led by big hospitals to fully accomplish the assignment of connecting the services between community medical care and big hospitals.

Supporting policies should also be in place. As for the global budget of 2021, the NHIA planned to use a fixed amount of 500 million NTD to guarantee that holiday and night outpatient visits in district hospitals are reimbursed at a fixed RVU value. The NHIA also explores the possibility of enhancing the capacity of district hospital services by providing measures such as: evaluating the upper limit for the number of support visits in district hospitals made by physicians from medical centers, regional hospitals and primary clinics, and encouraging the establishment of telemedicine models among hospitals of different levels, to strengthen people's confidence in community medical care.

Consolidate Small Hospitals in Remote Areas to Continuously Protect the Health of Residents

The main purpose of the implementation of NHI is to reduce the barriers to medical care for the disadvantaged; therefore, the NHIA especially focuses on those who reside in remote areas with scarce medical resources. And this is how the policy can intervene to assist hospitals that have established their foothold in remote areas to provide services continuously.

For hospitals established in mountainous areas, offshore islands, and areas with insufficient medical resources, or hospitals that are located in neighboring towns of the aforementioned areas, as long as they meet the requirements of the "Medical Service Improvement Plan for Areas with Insufficient Medical Resources" of the NHI, and provide 24-h emergency and outpatient services in Internal Medicine, Surgery, Obstetrics & Gynecology, and Pediatrics Departments, subsidies up to NTD 15 million each year would be granted to help these hospitals to have better medical delivery capabilities.

Co-Payment Adjustment

The spirit of the co-payment adjustment is not only to raise the public's cost awareness and let people cherish medical resources but also to further guide the correct medical behaviors of the insured, implement the tiered medical care system, and promote the separation of medicine and pharmacy. When unnecessary medical treatment is reduced, patients with minor illnesses and stable chronic diseases go to community institutions for medical treatment, and patients with acute and severe illnesses are referred to hospitals for treatment according to medical professions. The total amount of medical services will decrease, and the value of the RVUs will increase. The doctors have more time to take care of patients, and the quality of medical care will naturally improve, creating a win–win medical environment for patients and medical personnel. It promotes the efficiency of medical services, maximizes the benefits of health insurance, and achieves the goal of improving efficiency and quality through doctor–patient communication.

The NHIA refers to the opinions of all parties, analyzes the overall trend of the co-payment and the medical use situation, and proposes the following planning and thinking for reference and discussion. It is hoped that after the advice is widely accepted into the policy, a consensus can be gradually built, so that the public and medical service providers can accept and benefit.

Current Situation Analysis

There are two types of drug prescriptions: general drug prescriptions and continuous prescriptions for chronic diseases. According to the current collection analysis of the co-payments for drugs and examinations (tests), the average drug cost is NTD 381, but 70% of prescribed drugs are less than NTD 100, where the public does not have to bear the co-payments. Taking 2019 as an example, the NHI paid a total of NTD 80.6 billion for continuous prescriptions for chronic diseases, an average drug cost of NTD 985, but the public did not pay for any of them.

For examinations and tests, the average examination (test) cost per item is 1169 RVUs (1719 RVUs for medical centers, 1466 RVUs for regional hospitals, 1184 RVUs for district hospitals, and 435 RVUs for clinics). However, according to the current regulations, the co-payments of the examinations (tests) are not charged.

The Planning, Thinking, and Direction of Outpatient Co-Payments

With aging of the population, and the development of medical technology and new drugs, it is an indisputable fact that medical expenses have increased year by year. The number of RVUs claimed is much higher than the number approved, with the budgets falling into a vicious circle of doing more and getting less, making Taiwan known as a "sweat hospital." Further analysis shows that among the overall medical expenses, the annual increase in the cost of drugs and the examinations (tests) are the most obvious. Taking drugs as an example, there is no need to pay the co-payments for drugs under NTD 100 currently, and the maximum charges only NTD 200 for the drugs above NTD 1001. Some people took drugs home, but did not take them on time, causing a waste of resources. Furthermore, people do not need to pay extra costs for examinations or tests in hospitals, resulting in a small number of people who may ask doctors for additional examinations or tests.

The NHIA analyzed the suggestions of all parties comprehensively, planned adjustment measures for the co-payments, and focused on increasing the co-payments slightly, implementation of the tiered medical care system, and enhancement of the separation of medicine and pharmacy. The NHIA adopts a fixed-rate system to collect the costs that the people should bear in accordance with the NHIA, and also considers people's affordability and sets a ceiling price. It is hoped that with the paying part of the medical expenses, the people will think about whether to take more unnecessary drugs and do unnecessary tests, and the doctors should also carry out their responsibilities to inform patients about the necessity of the tests. It is hoped that the cost awareness of the people can be raised, the medical resources can be used appropriately, the insured can be further guided toward the correct behavior for medical care, and the tiered medical care system can be promoted continuously. The planning direction is divided into three parts: drugs, examination (tests), and emergency treatment.

1. Adjust the planning direction of co-payment for outpatient drugs:

   A. The NHIA plans to charge co-payments for outpatient drugs at a statutory rate and set a ceiling price. The plan to collect the co-payment of drugs for continuous prescriptions for chronic diseases is expected to improve the perception that patients with continuous prescriptions for chronic diseases do not cherish drugs because they do not have to bear the co-payment of drugs. However, it is still considered that patients with chronic diseases need long-term regular drugs, and there are concerns about the financial burden. Considering the amount that chronic patients need to bear, the co-payment at different levels of medical institutions and community pharmacies needs to be moderately adjusted.

   B. The NHIA will also plan to encourage people to go to district hospitals and clinics for medical treatment, and obtain drugs from community pharmacies, so as to implement the tiered medical care system and the separation of medicine and pharmacy.

2. The new planning direction of the co-payment for examinations (tests):

   A. The NHIA plans to charge the co-payments for examinations (tests) at a statutory rate. Considering that the issuance of examinations (tests) involves medical professional judgments, and the additional collecting of the co-payments will cause shocks in all walks of society and be more controversial. Therefore, people who cooperate with the tiered medical care system will be referred by a doctor after diagnosis and charged at a lower rate to the plan. After analysis, the average cost of each examination (test) at each level of medical institution is different, so different ceiling prices will be set according to the level and with or without referral.

   B. In addition, the NHIA will plan the co-payment mechanism for examinations (tests) toward the direction of encouraging people to go to district hospitals and clinics for medical care. If there are further medical needs, the primary doctors will refer patients to hospitals above the regional levels according to professional recommendations.

3. Adjust the planning direction of the co-payment for emergency care:

   When adjusting the co-payments of drugs and examinations (tests), the co-payments at the hospital level will approach or even exceed the quota for emergency care. It may cause people transfer to the emergency department for medical treatment. After investigation, the current emergency department does not collect the co-payments for drugs and examinations (tests), so the co-payments for the emergency department will be fine-tuned in coordination with the overall plan. We hope to advance the emergency medical resources of large hospitals to the tasks and roles of emergency and critical care, prevent mild cases from going to the emergency department of medical centers, and guide people toward behaving correctly in seeking medical care.

Conclusion

Providing a comprehensive and continuous service for people in Taiwan is always the aim of the NHI. With the ageing of the population and the development of medical care, medical expenses have increased year by year. To protect patients' medical rights with limited resources, expenditure reduction by inhibiting inappropriate use of medical resources is an answer to reduce the pressure of premium increases.

The high or low co-payments affect the rights and interests of most of those insured, because of Taiwan's medical convenience and the people's freedom of medical treatment. Our goal is to control the balance of interest conflicts and account for the rights of the insured and basic justice. The NHIA explains the concept and direction of the plans for everyone with reference and discussion. It is hoped that after the advice is widely accepted into the policy, a consensus can be gradually built, so that the public can accept and benefit.

References

1. Lih-Jen Lin, Shu-Ping Lee, 我國實施醫藥分業為何變雙軌制? The journal of Taiwan pharmacy, Volume 119, June 2014.
2. Min-Lang Chen, Limitations and Possibilities of the Praxis of Separation of Dispensing from Prescription. Journal of Social Sciences and Philosophy, Volume 23, Issue 4, July 2011; Kuo Shu-Ching, Implementation of Separation of Physician's dispensing, Master's Thesis of the Graduate Institute of National Policy and Public Affairs, NCHU, 1998.
3. 莊永明, 臺灣醫療史:以台大醫院為主軸, Yuan-Liou Publishing, June 1998

Chapter 5
Pursuing Health Equity

Po-Chang Lee, Yu-Chuan Liu, Yu-Hsuan Chang, Joyce Tsung-Hsi Wang,
Shu-Ching Chiang, and Hsueh-Yung Mary Tai

Introduction

The purpose of Taiwan National Health Insurance (NHI) is to improve the health
and secure the fairness of the medical rights of all citizens. To safeguard the health
of the disadvantaged, the National Health Insurance Administration (NHIA)
announced a full-scale unlocking of the NHI card to realize the universal right to
equal medical care. In addition, the NHIA conducted various programs that encourage providers to supply rural medical services, hoping to improve the accessibility
and comprehensiveness of medical care for residents of remote and offshore islands.
As for patients with rare diseases, the Legislative Yuan passed "The Rare Disease
and Orphan Drug Act" to offer more comprehensive care, making Taiwan the fifth
country in the world to protect the medical rights of patients with rare diseases
through legislation.

In addition to medical care for the disadvantaged, the health literacy of the public
is also the top priority of the NHIA. My Health Bank system enables users to query
their real-time medical and health information, which encourages self-health management and also improves the safety and quality of the medical care that they
receive. The NHI is introduced in elementary school textbooks to familiarize the
younger generation with its concept and create a more profound influence.

P.-C. Lee (✉) · Y.-C. Liu · J. T.-H. Wang · S.-C. Chiang · H.-Y. M. Tai
National Health Insurance Administration, Ministry of Health and Welfare, Taiwan,
Taipei, Taiwan
e-mail: pochang@nhi.gov.tw; B111262@nhi.gov.tw; mdjoyce@nhi.gov.tw;
grace7@nhi.gov.tw; marytai@nhi.gov.tw

Y.-H. Chang
Ministry of Health and Welfare, Taiwan, Taipei, Taiwan
e-mail: adsandychang@mohw.gov.tw

© The Author(s) 2022
P.-C. Lee et al. (eds.), *Digital Health Care in Taiwan*,
https://doi.org/10.1007/978-3-031-05160-9_5

Removing Barriers to Health Care to Protect the Disadvantaged

With the spirit of improving the health and safeguarding the fairness of medical rights of all citizens, the NHIA not only implements measures to assist the disadvantaged in paying the premium of the NHI but also gradually decouples the payment of premiums from the right to receive medical care for the disadvantaged (hereinafter referred to as unlocking of the NHI card) (Fig. 5.1). The number of people whose NHI card was locked owing to overdue NHI premiums dropped from 693,000 in 2007 to approximately 42,000 in April 2016. Furthermore, the NHIA announced a full-scale unlocking of the NHI card in June 2016 to realize the universal right to equal medical care, and to build a comprehensive umbrella to safeguard the health of the disadvantaged.

Decoupling of the Payment of Premiums from the Right to Receive Medical Care

To ensure the fair burden and the sustainability of the NHI, the public bear the responsibility of paying the premiums while enjoying the right to medical care. Therefore, the NHIA has a statutory disgorgement mechanism for those who owe

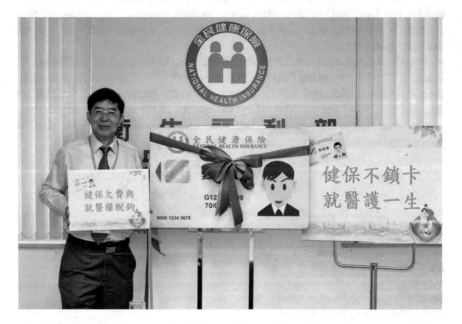

Fig. 5.1 Since June 2016, the policy of a full unlocking of the NHI card has been implemented

insurance premiums. The implementation of a full-scale unlocking of the NHI card means that no financially disadvantaged citizens will experience a delay in medical treatment because of their overdue premiums.

The NHIA combines the efforts from different sectors of the society and governmental agencies to assist the disadvantaged with premium payment and remove their psychological barriers when seeking medical treatment. Measures to provide those who are in need financially and care for the weakest in the society include (Fig. 5.2):

1. For low-income and middle-low-income households, the competent central social welfare authority subsidizes either all of or half their premiums respectively. The NHIA also acts as an agent to conduct subsidy projects from other government financial resources, including the premium subsidies for those who have physical and mental disabilities, and middle-low-income elderly aged 65–70 from each county and city government, the NHI premium subsidies for unemployed workers from the Bureau of Labor Insurance, and the NHI premium subsidies to new residents before their household registrations from the Ministry of the Interior.
2. Those who are unable to pay the premiums and overdue charges at one time owing to financial hardship may apply for an installment plan. For people with special circumstances, the NHIA approves a special installment plan that allows

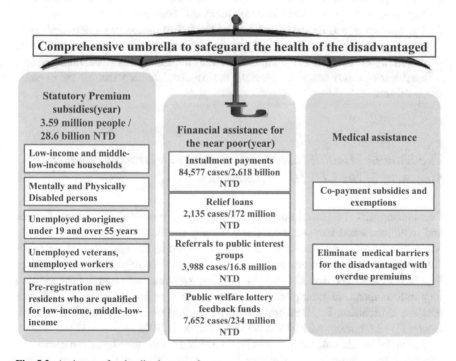

Fig. 5.2 Assistance for the disadvantaged

payment in up to 48 installments if the total annual individual income does not exceed personal exemption, standard deductions, and special deductions of income from salaries or wages for the most recent year.

3. Those who are qualify as financially difficult cases and who are unable to pay off the premiums may apply to the NHIA for an interest-free relief loan and start repaying from 1 year later. Eligible applicants include those who are legitimate middle-low-income households, and families whose main breadwinners suffer from major illnesses and injuries or who are unemployed for more than 6 months, etc.

4. The NHIA proposes the "Public Welfare Lottery Feedback Funds to Help the Disadvantaged to Defray Medical Expenses Plan" annually to obtain funding from the Ministry of Finance, to subsidize the premium of various financially disadvantaged groups.

5. The NHIA established a "Disadvantaged Notification Service Platform" that different sectors of the society can access to report information about cases that need assistance. The NHIA then connects external resources to assist the disadvantaged with their premiums by the NHI charity accounts, referrals to public interest groups, and public welfare lottery feedback funds.

6. For those who are financially disadvantaged with overdue premiums and meet the subject criteria of the Public Assistance Act (low-income households or middle-low-income elderly aged over 70), after confirming their inability to pay off the premiums, the NHIA will relieve their financial burden by not transferring their overdue premiums to compulsory enforcement.

7. The number of people applying for relief loans, installment payments, and referrals to public interest groups did not significantly decrease after the full-scale unlocking of the NHI card. This shows that the financially disadvantaged still need various assistance to alleviate the financial burden caused by overdue premiums.

The National Health Insurance Premium Deferment Paying Measures of the COVID-19 Epidemic

Considering that the global outbreak of COVID-19 may impact people's finance and livelihoods and hamper their ability to pay the NHI premiums on time, the NHIA allowed insured units and individuals affected by the pandemic to apply for deferment of their premium payments of February to July 2020 and April to September 2021. The overdue charges, payment reminder, and transfer for compulsory enforcement are exempted during the deferred period, so as to tide citizens over any difficulties. The total amount of the application is about New Taiwan dollars (NTD) 2.6 billion in 2020 and NTD 4.7 billion in 2021.

By the full-scale unlocking of the NHI card and all the assistance measures, the disadvantaged are no longer afraid of being unable to receive necessary medical care owing to overdue premiums. The move not only relieves their financial pressure and paves the last mile toward comprehensive protection to medical rights, but also helps to improve the health of all citizens and stabilize society. As for those who have the ability to repay, the NHIA continues to collect the arrears effectively and transfer them to compulsory enforcement, in order to avoid deliberate arrears and ensure that the full-scale unlocking of the NHI card does not impact the finance and operations of the NHI.

Medical Services on Remote and Offshore Islands

The NHI is committed to improving the accessibility and comprehensiveness of medical care for residents living on remote and offshore islands. With this goal in mind, the NHIA has carried out various initiatives since 1999 to encourage providers to invest in rural medical services, including the "Integrated Delivery System (IDS)," "Improvement Plan for Medically Underserved Areas," and "Upgrading Medical Services in Underserved Areas" plans, and others (Fig. 5.3). These initiatives are designed to incentivize more medical institutions and professionals to offer timely and affordable health care to under-resourced communities, with the full backing of the NHI system.

The Integrated Delivery System

The IDS coordinates and optimizes local medical resources, and provides diversified care appropriate to local conditions, including resident outpatient clinics, 24-h emergency services, night-time outpatient clinics, standby clinics for evenings and

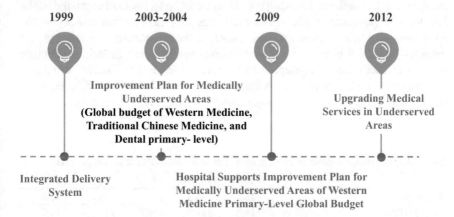

Fig. 5.3 The history of the National Health Insurance medical services promotion on remote and offshore islands

holidays, specialized medical care, specialized medical care bolstered by relevant medical staff, mobile clinic services, on-call medical services in the event of natural disasters, chronic disease management and prevention services, comprehensive home health care, and other medical services constituting a comprehensive network of care. Each IDS is unique to local conditions, implemented according to the distinctive needs of the community it services. Currently, there are 50 IDSs in full operation across Taiwan, buttressed by 26 large hospitals working in concert with local providers. In 2019 alone, the NHIA invested in a sum of NTD 5.04 billion in remote rural areas, of which IDS operations commanded NTD 1.17 billion. A total of 2012 specialist consultations were provided each month, serving more than 470,000 patients. From mountainous village clinics to offshore medical stations, IDS medical staff travel to wherever they are needed to provide high-quality, comprehensive health care to Taiwan's residents in remote areas.

In 2019, average visits per person in remote areas were 14.9 and 16.4 visits on offshore islands and mountain areas respectively. Notably, these averages were higher than that of the entire population (13.1 visits/person), of which a majority live on the main island, particularly in urban areas. Personal medical expenses in IDS areas were also comparable with those of the entire population (Tables 5.1 and 5.2). Since the program's inception in 1999, the IDS has attained a public satisfaction rate of more than 90%. The statistics above reflect gradually disappearing inequities in healthcare access and quality between highly populated urban areas and remote communities, as the NHIA looks beyond solely using IDS support to truly close the distance.

Improvement Plan for Medically Underserved Areas

Beyond deploying highly effective IDS networks across Taiwan, in order to mitigate inconvenience experienced seeking care in medically under-served areas, the NHIA has devised specialized initiatives to encourage medical professionals across the spectrum—traditional Chinese medicine doctors, Western medicine physicians, and dentists—to establish resident and mobile practices in areas still lacking adequate medical infrastructure. The Improvement Plan for Medically Underserved Areas was implemented in a total of 374 villages and towns in 2019 (Table 5.3), enabling an impressive 40,357 specialized consultations serving 710,144 patients.

Table 5.1 The average number of Western medicine outpatient visits per person per year

	2015	2016	2017	2018	2019
Mountain areas	16.1	16.3	16.3	16.1	16.4
Offshore islands	14.5	14.8	14.7	14.5	14.9
Entire population of the NHI insured	12.7	13.0	13.0	12.9	13.1

Unit: Times

Table 5.2 The average relative value units (RVUs) of Western medicine outpatient visits per person per year

	2015	2016	2017	2018	2019
Mountain areas	18,425	19,359	20,609	21,594	22,990
Offshore islands	13,824	14,518	15,672	16,472	17,325
Entire population of the NHI insured	14,943	15,650	16,565	17,409	18,261

Unit: RVUs
Source: The NHIA Data Warehouse system. People registered on the mountain areas and offshore islands and are insured, adjusted for age and gender
NHI = National Health Insurance

Table 5.3 Outcome of the Improvement Plan for Medically Underserved Areas for Western medicine, Traditional Chinese medicine, and dental in 2019

Sector of the global budget	Mobile health care			Rewarded practice
	Number of villages and towns	Total number of clinic (days)	Total person-times	Number of clinics
Hospitals	31	5023	67,884	–
Western medicine	83	12,598	236,030	13
Traditional Chinese medicine	111	11,174	278,599	2
Dental	149	11,562	127,631	28
Total	374	40,357	710,144	43

Upgrading Medical Services in Underserved Areas

To further enhance local healthcare services for residents in mountainous towns, offshore islands, and areas with insufficient medical resources, the "Upgrading Medical Services in Underserved Areas" initiative was implemented in 2012 to establish comprehensive health coverage in these communities, such as 24-h emergency services, inpatient services, as well as care spanning the disciplines of Internal Medicine, Surgery, Obstetrics and Gynecology, and Pediatrics. In total, 92 hospitals participated in providing needed care to underserved communities in 2019.

National Health Insurance Strives to Remove Barriers to Medical Treatment

The Kinmen IDS network implemented by the Taipei Division of the NHIA exemplifies the innovative work the NHIA has undertaken to remove all barriers to medical treatment, be them financial, economic, or geographical. The Taipei Veterans General Hospital (TVGH), as the pillar of the Kinmen IDS, deploys specialists to enhance the capabilities of Kinmen Hospital, so that major operations, such as craniotomy and cardiac catheterization, can now be performed in Kinmen. Patients suffering an ischemic stroke can receive thrombolytic therapy, and cancer patients can receive chemotherapy right on Kinmen Island—they and other Kinmen residents can rely on timely, potentially life-saving treatment without needing to travel to Taiwan's main island by boat.

Ms. Zhang, a Taiwanese citizen living abroad, was rescued from the grips of death by the IDS Kinmen team, an experience she shared on 17 December 2020, at a NHIA press conference reporting on the results of the Kinmen and Matsu IDS programs. Driving on a visit to Kinmen in July 2020, she encountered a serious car accident, which dealt her a traumatic intestinal injury, sternum fracture, chest contusion, blunt head injury, and severe laceration. Fortunately, the IDS medical team of Taipei Veterans General Hospital stationed at Kinmen Hospital, was available to give Ms. Zhang emergency life-saving treatment, afterward sending her to the TVGH main campus in Taipei for follow-up treatment. Ms. Zhang's full recovery from this otherwise fatal accident is one of many incredible testimonies to the importance of establishing equitable, comprehensive health care in remote and offshore areas.

Prospects

Beyond implementing an array of targeted, localized plans to improve the accessibility of no-compromise, high-quality medical services in remote and offshore areas, the NHIA ultimately aims to cultivate self-sustaining healthcare ecosystems in these areas. To this end, the NHIA leads efforts to recruit talents from a variety of specializations to provide resident services locally. A "National Physician Manpower Demand for Rural Areas Platform," featured on the homepage of the NHIA's official website, has been established to match physicians with fully reimbursed service opportunities in mountainous and offshore communities across the country. This platform is expected to foster a dynamic forum for mutual mentorship and progress, in which resident and visiting physicians learn from each other's experiences, in turn deepening the quality and longevity of health care in remote, under-resourced areas. At the same time, to avoid improper use of precious resources of the National Health Insurance and ensure the quality of medical services in underserved communities, the NHIA continues to monitor the service capacities and perform on-site visits to assess the quality of the on-the-ground services delivered by both resident clinics and mobile stations alike, and regulates hospitals that deviate from the central goal of serving still under-resourced communities, e.g., by fraudulently claiming compensation.

National Health Insurance Stands by Patients with Rare Diseases

To care for patients with rare diseases more comprehensively, the Legislative Yuan passed "The Rare Disease and Orphan Drug Act" in 2000. In the past two decades, the NHI has served as the patients' strongest support. As of 2019, there are 9600 rare-disease patients receiving drugs covered by the NHI.

Rare diseases are uncommon diseases with a low prevalence rate, and according to "The Rare Disease and Orphan Drug Act" the definition of "rare disease" is "diseases with prevalence lower than the standard announced by the central competent authority (1 in 10,000)." Under special circumstances, a disease could be recognized as a rare disease through review by the Review Committee for Rare Diseases and Orphan Drugs (hereafter referred to as the Review Committee) and designated and publicly announced by the central competent authority. Orphan drugs are used to prevent, diagnose, and treat rare diseases, under the premise of being recognized through review by the Review Committee and announced by the central competent authority. The same Act also stipulates that after obtaining designation or special approval from the central competent authority, orphan drugs can be submitted for listing in the National Health Insurance Pharmaceutical Benefits and Reimbursement Scheme. As of the end of December 2020, the NHI covered 207 drug items that had either been announced by the competent authority as drugs eligible for special importation (manufacture) or those qualified for orphan drug licenses under the Rare Disease and Orphan Drug Act.

Rare Diseases Are Categorized as Catastrophic Illnesses to Waive Patient Co-Payments

Given that patients with rare disease are uncommon, they have higher and more urgent medical needs owing to the severity of their health conditions, the NHIA has classified all individuals with rare diseases as having catastrophic illness. In this way, their co-payments for medical care could be waived, reducing the heavy financial burden of families with a member who has a rare disease. As of the end of May 2020, the Ministry of Health and Welfare has announced a total of 223 categories of rare diseases. According to the statistics in 2019, the largest number of patients with rare diseases who applied for a catastrophic illness certificate comprises multiple sclerosis patients with brain or nervous system lesions, a total of 1445 patients (Table 5.4).

The NHIA has always been very concerned about the medical rights of patients with rare diseases. Since 2005, it has strived for a dedicated budget for orphan drugs to avoid rare-disease cases from being squeezed out by the Global Budget owing to the high medical expenses. Expenditures for orphan drugs increased from 1.738 billion RVUs in 2010 to 6.167 billion RVUs in 2019, and the average growth rate of

Table 5.4 Number of patients with rare diseases applying for the ten most common catastrophic illness certificates

Ranking	Rare disease	2017	2018	2019
1	Multiple sclerosis	1395	1250	1445
2	Spinocerebellar ataxia	916	921	935
3	Tuberous sclerosis	562	589	624
4	Amyotrophic lateral sclerosis	562	564	562
5	Wilson's disease	513	515	536
6	Achondroplasia	386	393	399
7	Spinal muscular atrophy	366	375	388
8	Primary pulmonary hypertension	309	315	346
9	Charcot–Marie–Tooth	278	308	312
10	Thalassemia major	316	313	337
Other diseases		5432	6002	6269
Total		**11,035**	**11,545**	**12,153**

annual cost in the past 5 years is about 11.2%. We further analyzed the medical resource utilization of various rare diseases. Taking 2019 as an example, patients who contributed the highest average drug costs are those with mucopolysaccharidoses (9.938 million RVUs per patient), followed by Gaucher's disease and Fabry's disease (9.832 million RVUs per patient and 7.753 million RVUs per patient respectively).

Because of the scarcity of patients with rare diseases, the pharmaceutical companies are often unwilling to invest in the development of drugs for rare diseases owing to the economic scale. As a consequence, production costs and unit prices for rare-disease drugs are extremely high. Without alternative treatments on the market, the drugs for rare diseases are also called "orphan drugs." In response to patients' demand, the NHIA proactively includes orphan drugs in its benefit package. For example, Spinraza, a drug for the treatment of spinal muscular atrophy (SMA), has been covered by the NHI since 1 July 2020. This not only brings good news to patients, but also starts a new page for NHI's coverage for SMA treatments.

Strengthening Control Measures for Orphan Drugs

However, considering that the medical expenses of rare diseases have increased year by year recently, the NHIA has begun to strengthen control over orphan drugs. Starting from 1 September 2019, only patients with rare diseases recognized by the Health Promotion Administration are eligible for orphan drugs. It is hoped that with assistance from medical institutions, patients with rare diseases could obtain their catastrophic illness certificates promptly. By doing so, their financial burden could be reduced or eliminated, and they could qualify for using orphan drugs and be treated properly.

Another control measure is the routine review for the prices of orphan drugs. According to Article 24 of the Regulations on Drug Price Adjustment of the NHI, the payment for orphan drugs should be reviewed and adjusted every 2 years. In addition, Article 35, Item 2 of the "National Health Insurance Pharmaceutical Benefit and Reimbursement Scheme" also stipulates: "Orphan drugs included in this scheme without drug license must acquire drug license or documents certifying their safety and efficacy from the competent authority within 3 years, or they will be subject to delisting. However, drugs that have obtained the US or EU market approval are exempt from this requirement, and their prices may be reduced by 5% annually." The NHIA will continue to collect opinions from experts and scholars and revise the orphan drug payment regulations according to clinical evidence. For example, the review of the orphan drugs payment for mucopolysaccharidoses and Fabry's disease was carried out and implemented in December 2018 and September 2019 respectively. In addition to the abovementioned policies, we will evaluate the efficacy of high-priced orphan drugs constantly in the future to ensure the rational allocation of NHI resources.

Changes in health status are often unpredictable. The offspring of healthy persons may also be at risk of suffering from rare diseases. Therefore, the NHIA always treats patients and their families with empathy. Life is valuable for everyone to pursue their own opportunities. Even though the medical expenses of patients with rare diseases are high, we uphold the spirit of caring for the disadvantaged and allocate limited resources fairly. In consideration of medical rights, fairness and justice, and social ethics, we firmly support patients with rare diseases by fulfilling medical needs that their lives depend on. We call on everyone to cherish medical resources together, so that every dollar of the premium of the NHI contributed by each citizen can benefit more insured people in need of medical care.

My Health Bank—Promoting Self-Health Management

My Health Bank Guards Our Health

To realize "people-centered health care," the NHIA applied the concept of My Data to establish "My Health Bank" in 2014. People can browse their medical and health information of the past 3 years on their mobile devices, including outpatient records, inpatient records, surgical data, medication records, allergy data, examination and test results, imaging and pathological examination, test reports, hospital discharge summaries, willingness for organ donation, hospital palliative care, adult preventive care, vaccination records, physiological measurement, hepatoma risk prediction, evaluation of end-stage renal disease and other information. Possessing personal health records not only encourages their self-health management but helps them to communicate with medical providers, and thereby improves the safety and quality of the medical care they receive.

Rapid Cell Phone-Based Certification Allows Users to Manage Their Medical Information Easily

The NHIA integrated personal health information of "My Health Bank" into "National Health Insurance Mobile Easy Access" mobile application (NHI Express app). The function of rapid cell phone-based certification for users' identity was further added in May 2018 under the premise of information security. The rapid cell phone-based certification function of the NHI Express app makes it the first application that government agencies use on a large scale for identity certification through cell phones because of its safety and convenience.

To allow people to search information related to the National Health Insurance quickly in a more intuitive and user-friendly way, the NHIA continues to optimize the operation surface and the service process of the NHI Express app. A modified vision was introduced in March 2021, aiming to enhance the quality and efficiency of these convenience services.

Family Member Management Function Added to Safeguard Family Health

The family member management function was added to the My Health Bank system in May 2019. For the elderly and children under 15 who are less familiar with electronic products, a designated person can access the My Health Bank system for the elderly and children on his or her own cell phone through the family member management function to assist their health management (Fig. 5.4).

Software Development Kit Connects Health Services Better

To further apply the use of the My Health Bank system to more diversified settings, the NHIA developed the Software Development Kit (SDK) of the My Health Bank system in May 2019, so that third-party apps can connect with the My Health Bank system through the SDK. After authorization, users can select personal medical treatment, medication, test results and other information within a specific period in the My Health Bank system freely, download and store it on mobile devices and bridge it to trusted third-party apps. The third-party apps can combine their original functions with medical information so that the user can receive more value-added healthcare services, such as online medical consultation, chronic disease management, while using the apps they are already accustomed to. The data from the My Health Bank system integrated to the third-party app enhances the completeness and value of health information, and therefore makes it easier for its user to manage their health.

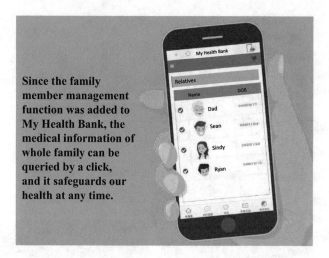

Since the family member management function was added to My Health Bank, the medical information of whole family can be queried by a click, and it safeguards our health at any time.

Fig. 5.4 Family member management function safeguards our family's health

As of 9 November 2021, a total of 130 manufacturers (306 apps) have applied, 23 of which (47 apps) have been officially launched. Among them, 11 are health information management software companies, 9 are medical institutions, 2 are medicine and medical device manufacturers, and 1 is a government agency.

Supporting Name-Based Mask Distribution System to Assist the Country in Epidemic Prevention

The global pandemic of COVID-19 continued to heat up in 2020. The name-based mask distribution system was implemented in February 2020 to ensure a stable supply of anti-epidemic masks, granting people equal opportunities to purchase masks, and the NHI card was used as the ID for purchasing masks at pharmacies. The name-based mask distribution system 2.0 was implemented in March of the same year and the NHI Express app is utilized for mask preorder processing, and a review of purchase history. In this way, purchasing masks is much easier for populations such as office workers and students so that they no longer have to wait in a long queue at pharmacies.

The function of the My Health Bank system also continues to increase. The total number of medical visits and a detailed history of medical visits were added to the system (Fig. 5.5). By displaying the total number of medical visits in each of the past 3 years, as well as the number of RVUs claimed by medical institutions and co-payments paid, we look forward to helping the public to understand and cherish the resources of the NHI overall (Fig. 5.6).

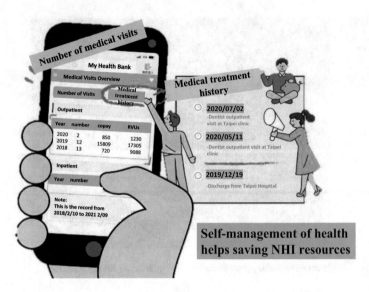

Fig. 5.5 My Health Bank—overview function of medical visits

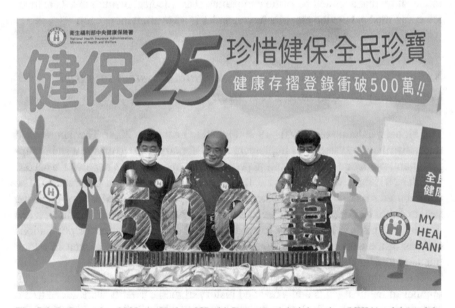

Fig. 5.6 In September 2020, the National Health Insurance Administration (NHIA) celebrated the 25th anniversary of the National Health Insurance and over 5 million logins to My Health Bank. Premier Su Tseng-Chang, Health Minister Chen Shih-Chung, and NHIA Director General Lee declared the opening of the ceremony together. (From Executive Yuan. https://www.ey.gov.tw/Page/AF73D471993DF350/a3b1039f-ad86-4571-a713-f2cb7eb986cb)

The Significance of Including National Health Insurance in Elementary School Teaching Materials

It has been 27 years since the inception of the NHI in 1995. If we personify the life course of the NHI, it is already a college graduate who has entered the workforce. However, even though many people rely on the NHI, their understanding of it is still at the "kindergarten" level. Some people think the NHI is just like private medical insurance, life insurance, and accident insurance; some people think that because they pay the NHI premium every month, it is a waste not to use it and even want to earn their money back; some people think that the NHI will take care of them when they are sick anyway, so they neglect their obligation to take care of their own health. Therefore, we hope that pupils can understand the meaning and value of the NHI through the articles and lectures in the elementary school Chinese curriculum to cultivate the concept of cherishing the NHI resources in the younger generation.

When organ donation was actively promoted at National Cheng Kung University Hospital, an organ recipient Mr. Chao-jung Huang wrote about his life experience in an article "Love Doesn't Die." After being rewritten by the National Institute for Compilation and Translation and Hanlin Publishing Company, the article was included in the fifth-grade textbook. When promoting a concept with activities such as field trips or speeches, the audience reached is limited because of time and space constraints. However, by integrating the concept into textbooks that are read by tens of thousands of students every year, the idea takes root from generation to generation, creating a more profound influence.

The establishment of the concept of the NHI must start at an early age. By incorporating it into elementary school textbooks, the concept can be conveyed from teachers to students, from students to their families, and then spread from close family members to other relatives and neighboring communities. The NHIA has always emphasized and promoted the value of "cherishing the resources of the NHI." Officials of the NHIA visited the Ministry of Education to explain this idea in person. The Minister of Education, Wen-chung Pan, also recognized further incorporating the concept of the NHI into education (Fig. 5.7). Both disciplines of Health and Physical Education and Society in the 9th year and the 12th year include related topics such as understanding of the NHI and medical system and avoiding resource abuse.

By introducing and discussing the social phenomena presented in the texts, teachers can gradually foster students' sense of citizenship. Although the two subjects of Health and Physical Education and Society touch upon the concept of the NHI, the Chinese course, for 5 h per week, allows children to have more time for reading and thinking. Therefore, the ultimate goal is to include the NHI in a Chinese subject textbook.

The NHIA has visited several publishers to discuss these ideas. As Hanlin Publishing Company has adapted the article describing the experience of organ donation, "Love Doesn't Die," it highly recognizes the educational concept of the

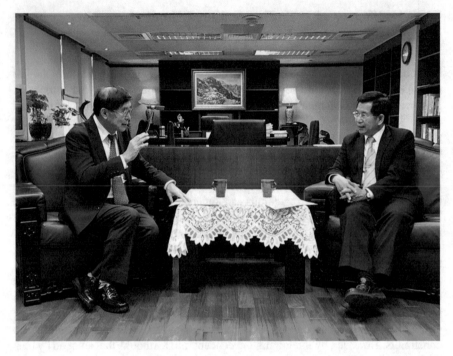

Fig. 5.7 On 15 December 2017, Director Po-Chang Lee visited with Minister of Education Wen-chung Pan

NHIA, and strongly supports including it in Chinese subject textbooks. After many discussions, Hanlin assisted in the drafting of "The Most Admired Health Care System in Asia" and included it in the "Reading Paradise" unit of the fifth-grade Chinese subject textbook. In addition, Nani Publishing also promised to include two articles about the NHI in the Chinese subject workbook of the fifth grade in elementary school, so that children can also be exposed to the concept of the NHI when practicing new words learned in the class (Table 5.5).

In these textbook articles, Ms. Shu-chu Chen's childhood experience is used to illuminate that because of the medical care provided by the NHI, no Taiwanese are unable to seek medical treatment owing to economic barriers. We also mention the current development of information technology and provide students with a preliminary understanding of the convenience brought about by the "National Health Insurance MediCloud System (NHI MediCloud System)," so that they can have more confidence in tiered medical care. The functions and advantages of "My Health Bank" are introduced to strengthen the ability of self-care. The most precious thing is using this opportunity to explain the spirit of "mutual assistance" of the NHI with easy-to-understand wording and inspire both older and younger readers to internalize the concept of cherishing the resources of the NHI.

Table 5.5 The topic of National Health Insurance is included in Chinese elementary school textbooks

Publisher	Items of teaching materials	Descriptions	Schedule
Hanlin	Textbooks, workbooks, teacher manuals	1. There is one article in the textbook of the second semester of the fifth grade: "The Most Admired Health Care System in Asia" 2. Compiling workbooks and teacher manuals in line with textbooks, and there are four related articles in teacher manuals: 　A. "Healthy life is the happiest" by Children's literature writer Wen ya Gui 　B. "Invisible Pride" by Deputy Director of the NHIA Planning Division Fu-Chung Wang 　C. "Guardian Angel of Lanyu" by Dr. Chia-Hsuan Wu 　D. "Classmates said" by Associate Professor Yao-Mao Chang	Available from the second semester of the 2019 academic year (February 2020)
Nani	Workbooks	There are two articles in the workbooks of the first semester of the fifth grade, which are compiled in the phonetic notation of Chinese characters to fill in the blanks, so that students can be exposed to the concept of the National Health Insurance while reviewing the new words learned in this lesson	Available from the first semester of the 2019 academic year (September 2019)
Kang Hsuan	Teacher manuals	One article in the Appendix of the teacher manuals of the first semester of the second grade, containing the article of the NHIA interview with Ms. Chen Shu-chu "the National Health Insurance is life-saving money for taking care of everyone's health," is provided for teachers' reference as needed when teaching	Available from the first semester of the 2018 academic year (September 2018)

The incorporation of the concept of the NHI into Chinese subject textbooks was carried out in 2020. We believe that the goal of cultivating the concept of cherishing the NHI resources in the general public will be achieved step by step from now on (Table 5.6).

Table 5.6 The content of the elementary Chinese subject textbook about Taiwan's National Health Insurance published by Hanlin Publishing Company (From Hanlin Publishing Company. https://www.hle.com.tw/index.html)

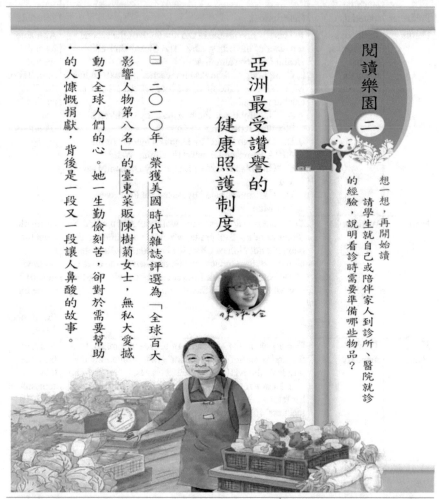

The Most Admired Health Care System in Asia	**Reading Paradise 2**
Author: Su-Ling Chen	Try to answer the question before
A vegetable vendor in Taitung, Ms. Shu-Chu Chen, was	you start reading.
ranked as the eighth place among the top 100 influential	Please describe what items are
people in the world by American Time Magazine in 2010, as	needed when you visit a clinic or
her selflessness moved people all over the world. She has	hospital by yourselves or
been hardworking and thrifty all her life, but generously	accompanied by your family
donated to those in need. However, there are several sad	members.
stories behind her kindness.	

(continued)

Table 5.6 (continued)

陳樹菊女士在十三歲時，因為家裡貧困，湊不出給醫院的五千元保證金，導致母親因延遲送醫而難產過世；後來，她的三弟突然生了一場怪病，家裡一時間湊不出醫療費，錯過最佳搶救時機而回天乏術。即便事隔多年，陳樹菊女士每每憶起這些往事，還是忍不住紅了眼眶：「因為我們太窮了，如果我們有錢的話，家人就不會因為湊不齊醫藥費而離開……」這是陳樹菊女士家中既悲慘又無奈的真實故事，也是那個沒有健保制度的年代裡，許多貧困家庭的類似寫照——有病無錢醫。

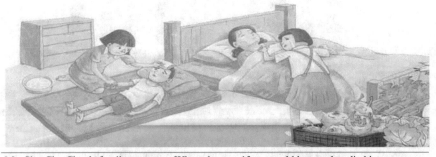

Ms. Shu-Chu Chen's family was poor. When she was 13 years old her mother died in childbirth because her family couldn't make up the NTD 5000 deposit for the hospital. Later on, her third brother suddenly had an unknown disease. Her family missed the best time to rescue him and lost him because they couldn't make up the medical expenses immediately. Even after many years, Ms. Chen Shu-Chu couldn't help but fill her eyes whenever she recalled these memories: "Because we were too poor. If we had money, our family member would not have left us. It was because we could not come up with money for medical expenses..." This is the true story from Ms. Chen Shu-Chu's miserable and helpless family. It is also a portrait of many poor families in the era when there was no health insurance system—they did not have savings or the means to pay for the medical care they needed.

(continued)

Table 5.6 (continued)

（三）曾經苦過，才真正明白苦的滋味。陳樹菊女士因此願意無償為「全

民健康保險」代言，在健保，有你真好的短片中，她有感而發的說：

「以前生病沒有健保，都要去跟別人借錢，……那種沒錢救命的艱苦，

等你遇到，你就知道。」的確，如果沒有經歷過「沒錢救命的艱苦」，

確實很難真正體會。身處臺灣當今完善健保制度下的國民，我們應該對

全民健康保險有更多的認識與支持。

全民健康保險標誌

（四）拿出健保卡，你可以在晶片上方，發現有個圓形標誌，標誌中間有

兩個「小綠人」，這可不是協助我們過馬路的小綠人交通號誌，而是

「全民健康保險標誌」呵！仔細瞧瞧，標誌以一男一女握手表示「互相

Only those who have suffered understand the taste of bitterness. Therefore, Ms. Shu-Chu Chen is willing to endorse the NHI for free. In the short film "It's nice to have the National Health Insurance," she said with sentiment: "When there was no National Health Insurance you had to borrow money from others when you get sick, …… you won't understand the hardships of no money for saving lives until you encounter it." Indeed, if you haven't experienced the hardships, it is difficult to truly understand. We Taiwanese enjoying the comprehensive health insurance system now should know more about and support the National Health Insurance.

Logo of the National Health Insurance

You can find a circular logo on the top of the NHI card. There are two "little green persons" in the middle of the logo. It is not the little green man traffic sign that helps us to cross the road, but a logo of the NHI! Take a closer look, the logo shows a man and a woman shaking hands, which means:

(continued)

Table 5.6 (continued)

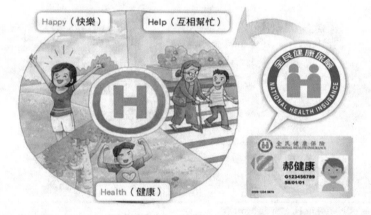

幫助、互相照顧，大家都健康」的意思。再進一步聯想，這個男女握手圖案很像哪個英文字母？沒錯，就像英文字母「H」！你知道嗎？這個「H」隱含三個特殊的意義呵！分別是互相幫忙（Help）、健康（Health）、快樂（Happy），也就是說：「如果大家都能互相幫忙，就能健康又快樂！」這個標誌，是不是很有意思，也很有意義呢？

"Help each other and take care of each other, and then everyone will be healthy." Let's further imagine, which English letter does this male and female shaking hands pattern look like? Yes, it's the English letter "H"! Do you know? This "H" implies three special meanings, which are "Help" each other, "Health," and "Happy." It means that: "If everyone helps each other, everyone can be healthy and happy!" Isn't this sign very interesting and meaningful?

(continued)

Table 5.6 (continued)

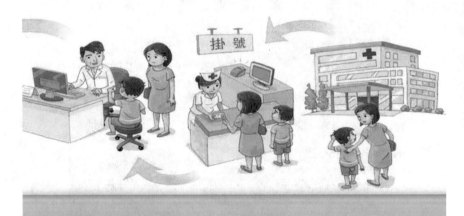

全民健康保險的特色

Help 互相幫忙，關懷弱勢

（五）

由「Help」的意義來說，全民
健康保險是「強制性」的保險，自
一九九五年開辦以來，健保費收入主
要來自民眾、雇主及政府共同分擔。
更值得一提的是，自二〇一六年六月
起，健保署讓積欠健保費的人，必要
時也可以及時就醫，以減少像陳樹菊
女士的親人一樣，因為經濟困頓，無
法順利就醫而造成的終身遺憾；同時

Features of National Health Insurance

Help

Help each other and care for the disadvantaged

Let's start form the meaning of "Help." The National Health Insurance is a compulsory program. Since its inception in 1995, the insurance has been financed mainly by the premium contribution of the public, employers, and the government. It is worth mentioning that the NHIA has allowed people who owe premiums to seek medical treatment in time when necessary, since June 2016. The purpose is to prevent life-long regrets just like Ms. Chen Shu-Chu's relatives, who were unable to go to the doctor owing to financial difficulties.

(continued)

Table 5.6 (continued)

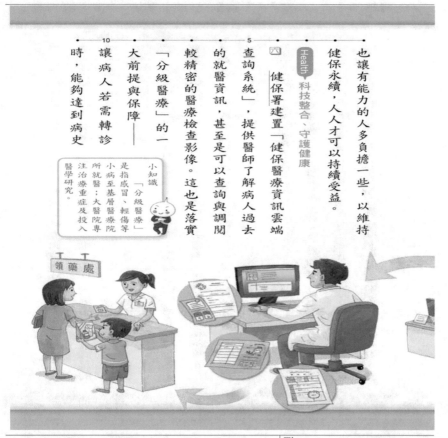

At the same time, it also allows better-off people to contribute more to maintain the sustainability of the National Health Insurance and benefits everyone continuously.

Health

Technology integration safeguards our health

The NHIA has built the National Health Insurance MediCloud System to provide physicians with patients' medical information and access to more sophisticated medical examination images. This is also a major prerequisite and guarantee for the implementation of the "tiered medical care system"—if the patient needs to be referred, the medical history information can be exchanged smoothly. Everyone can also obtain his or her medical and medication records within the past 3 years by checking their "My Health Bank" online, and fully understand their personal health status. It is a good aid to self management of health!

Tips

In the "tiered medical care system," treatment of minor illnesses such as colds and minor injuries are taken care of in clinics; large hospitals focus on treating severe illnesses and contributing to medical research.

(continued)

Table 5.6 (continued)

資訊暢通無礙。每個人也可以透過網路查詢「健康存摺」，了解自己三

年內的就醫及用藥等紀錄，掌握個人健康狀況等，是自我健康管理的好

幫手呢！

> Happy 全民滿意、身心愉悅

臺灣全民健康保險制度以「互相照顧、互相幫忙」的良善理念為出

發點，集合眾人的力量，落實平等就醫的權利，近年來滿意度維持在八

成以上。人們能因健保獲得完整持續的醫療照護，擁有健康的身體，進

一步擁有快樂的身心。

全民健康保險讓臺灣被世界讚賞

（四）二○○八年美國公共電視網製作了專題報導，比較英國、臺灣、

德國、瑞士和日本等五個國家的醫療保險制度，讚揚臺灣的健康照護服

務、智慧型健保卡、醫療照護費用不及美國一半等優勢，都成為探討焦

> Happy

All people are satisfied, feeling happy inside out

Taiwan's National Health Insurance system is based on the concept of goodness: "care for each other and help each other." It aggregates the power of everyone to realize the goal of providing equal rights to medical care. In recent years, more than 80% of people surveyed are satisfied with the service of the National Health Insurance. The comprehensive and continuous medical care provided by the National Health Insurance contributes to healthy bodies, and further brings physical and mental wellness.

Taiwan is widely recognized by the world for its National Health Insurance

In 2008, the US Public Broadcasting Service produced a special report that compared the health insurance systems of five countries, including the United Kingdom, Taiwan, Germany, Switzerland, and Japan. The report praised Taiwan's healthcare services, smart NHI cards, and low medical costs, which are less than half of those in the United States. These strengths have all become the focus of discussion.

(continued)

Table 5.6 (continued)

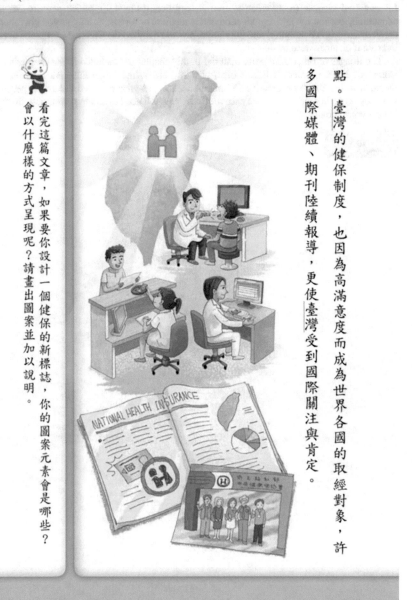

After reading this article, if you want to design a new logo for the National Health Insurance, what will your elements be? In what way will it be presented? Please draw the pattern and explain it.

Taiwan's National Health Insurance system has also become the model for countries around the world because of its high satisfaction rate. Various reports from international media and journals brought Taiwan more attention and affirmation from people around the world.

Chapter 6
Infrastructure of the Medical Information System

Hsueh-Yung (Mary) Tai and Shwu-Huey Wu

Introduction

Since the launch of the National Health Insurance (NHI) in 1995, people in Taiwan can receive healthcare properly and conveniently without barriers, and their medical rights are also protected. People only need to afford the registration fee and a small amount of co-payment to seek medical care. In 2019, the total number of outpatient visits was 367.61 million, which was equivalent to 1 million visits per day, and the average number of outpatient visits per person per year is much higher than that of Organization for Economic Cooperation and Development member countries.

To process medical claims submitted by NHI-contracted medical institutions, the NHIA established medical information systems. Coupled with the NHI IC card launched in 2004, the National Health Insurance entered a new era of comprehensive informatization. The application of the NHI virtual private network (VPN) and centralized information system enables contracted medical institutions to fully digitalize claims. Platforms such as the National Health Insurance MediCloud System (NHI MediCloud System) were constructed to encourage medical providers to share medical examination reports, test reports, and images promptly.

H.-Y. (Mary) Tai (✉) · S.-H. Wu
National Health Insurance Administration, Ministry of Health and Welfare,
Taipei, Taiwan
e-mail: marytai@nhi.gov.tw; shwu@nhi.gov.tw

© The Author(s) 2022
P.-C. Lee et al. (eds.), *Digital Health Care in Taiwan*,
https://doi.org/10.1007/978-3-031-05160-9_6

Cornerstone of the National Health Insurance Database— Introduction to the NHI Medical Information System

The NHIA medical information system is constructed mainly for internal and external medical business services. The NHI Intranet, which enables officers of the NHIA to execute various healthcare affairs of the NHI, applies a multi-tier architecture and the actual information data center are located in Taipei and Taichung to back each other up. Externally, the medical information system provides the NHI applications system (including VPN and Internet) for medical institutions, pharmaceutical companies, special medical device suppliers, and the general public to carry out relevant healthcare services. The overall operating environment runs on a well-protected network of the NHI and the relevant system architecture diagram is shown Fig. 6.1.

Highly Automated Process of Medical Claims

The medical information system mainly processes the claim submission, acceptance, and data verification of the medical claims. Administrative review is a series of automated reviews conducted by computers, followed by sampling and professional peer review, and then an accounting and approval procedure. Except for professional peer review, the main medical claim process has been highly automated to improve the efficiency of the operation and the consistency of claim data verification, so that the medical reimbursement can be finalized within 60 days after acceptance.

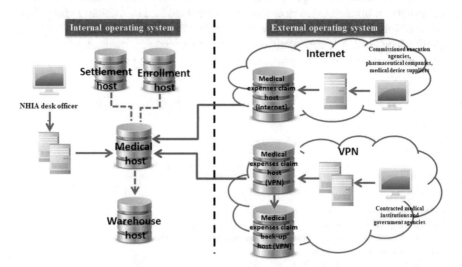

Fig. 6.1 Medical information system architecture diagram

In addition to the basic medical claim data, the system also collects relevant data that formulate through medical pilot projects by the NHIA and daily uploading NHI IC card medical information from contracted medical institutions to conduct various service-related inspections. The NHIA also undertakes commissioned business from other government agencies. For example, the Health Promotion Administration (HPA) entrusts the NHIA with paying medical expenses for various preventive health care, and the Bureau of Labor Insurance entrusts the payment of medical expenses for occupational injuries. Owing to the condition of the entrusted businesses, the system, structures, and requirements of information for data editing, accounting, and payment approval procedures are different.

The medical information system mainly functions as an operational environment for internal medical claims and reviews and it also provides an external web service platform for contracted medical institutions, pharmaceutical companies, and special medical device suppliers to submit and obtain the results of claims data. The medically related data are uploaded into the NHI Data Warehouse information system regularly for subsequent statistical analysis and decision-making assistance applications. The main process of the medical system is shown in Fig. 6.2.

In response to the increasing number of claims that required professional peer review, and to provide a timely and remote cross-regional review function, the NHIA has constructed and upgraded related equipment to establish a centralized medical images system, the Picture Archiving and Communication System, hoping to lay a solid foundation for precise reviews.

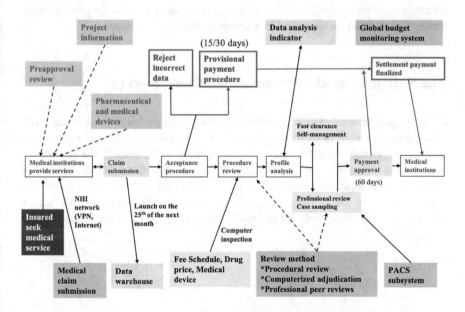

Fig. 6.2 The main process of the medical information system

Establishing National Health Insurance MediCloud System
to Implement a Tiered Medical Care System

In recent years, the NHIA has been actively constructing the NHI MediCloud System to encourage medical institutions to upload medical examination reports and images promptly and expand the scope of digital review. At the same time, the NHIA also incentivizes medical institutions to establish a two-way referral mechanism under the tiered medical care system through various programs. Meanwhile, the NHIA strengthens the integration function of the "Intelligent Peer Review System." This effort included the establishment of automatic links to health insurance payment regulations, review guidelines, patient's electronic medical records, reviews of focal point information, reminder mechanisms and individualized settings in helping medical reviewers to perform their work accurately and efficiently. The NHIA further integrates the artificial intelligence (AI) analysis module of the Data Warehouse system and give feedback to doctors as a reference, so as to improve the accuracy of professional review and the efficiency of the peer review process.

The NHIA has carried out a number of medical policy reforms according to important national healthcare guidelines, and the implementation of these policies requires a powerful information system as its foundation. With rapid changes and developments in different stages of the medical policy, the NHIA needs to modify relevant medical information systems to keep up with the changes accordingly to accommodate rapid developments of information technology and guarantee operation efficiency and information security simultaneously. To enhance medical services of the NHI, the Information Management Division of the NHIA endeavors to maintain smooth operation of the medical information system, to provide high-quality information services, and to accomplish missions assigned.

The National Health Insurance MediCloud System

Many people are used to seeking medical care in different hospitals or visiting different doctors owing to different illnesses, so their personal medical records and medication history are scattered in different medical institutions. When doctors can hardly view patients' previous medical records from other medical institutions promptly, then duplicated medications can be provided and examinations or tests can be conducted easily. Drug–drug interactions caused by duplicated medication may affect medication safety for patients, and also may result in the waste of medical resources.

Building Patient-Centered "NHI PharmaCloud System"

The NHIA built a patient-centered "NHI PharmaCloud System" by using computing technology in July 2013. This system provided assembled patients' recent medication records by consolidating medical claims data from medical institutions and data uploaded via the NHI IC card. To avoid duplicated medications and enhance drug safety for patients, this system allows doctors and pharmacists to view patients' medication records.

Upgrading of the "NHI MediCloud System"

The NHIA upgraded the "NHI PharmaCloud System" into the "NHI MediCloud System" in 2015. When doctors are providing clinical treatments and/or prescriptions or pharmacists are dispensing medicines and/or providing medical consultations, they can access the NHI MediCloud System to query 12 categories of patient medical records, such as western and traditional Chinese medication records, examination records and results, surgery records, dental care records, drug allergy records, specific medication records of controlled drugs and coagulation factors, rehabilitation records, discharge summary and vaccination records from the Centers of Disease Control (CDC) (Fig. 6.3).

In 2018, medical images such as computed tomography (CT), magnetic resonance imaging (MRI), X-ray, ultrasound, gastroscopy, and colonoscopy can be uploaded and shared in the NHI MediCloud System (Fig. 6.4), thus allowing doctors to obtain patients' medical information in real time in different medical institutions.

In May 2018, the NHIA expanded the one-way provision of patients' medical information to a two-way information exchange model, so that medical professionals can report "drug therapeutic inequivalence," "questionable quality of uploaded medical images," and "drug allergy" to the NHI MediCloud System to improve the efficiency of information sharing and the quality of medical services.

Design of Active Reminders in the NHI MediCloud System

To increase efficiency and effort in browsing plenty of information and enhancing safety, "active reminder for duplicated orders" and "active reminder for drug interactions and/or allergies" have been provided since September 2018. By instant comparison with the NHI database, these functions remind doctors if there are duplicated orders, drug–drug interactions upon patients' remaining medicine, or drug allergies when medicine or treatment codes are entered into the Hospital Information System (HIS) from prescriptions.

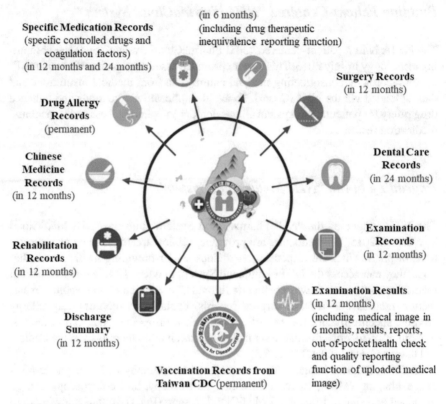

Fig. 6.3 Functions of the NHI MediCloud System

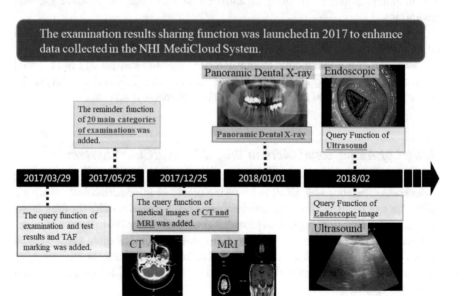

Fig. 6.4 Development of medical images uploading and sharing

Personal Privacy Protection and Information Security Management

Because medical information is highly private and sensitive, since the initiation of the NHI PharmaCloud System, the NHIA has gathered professionals from relevant fields such as information, medical quality management, and law to jointly discuss system settings, regulations on the use of medical institutions, etc.

1. Establishing the Authentication Mechanism and Management for Data Acquisition

   The system is built in a closed VPN, in which only when three necessary cards, i.e., the medical institution secure access module card, physician card (or pharmacist card), and the patients' NHI IC card, are verified during the visit can healthcare providers obtain patients' medical history. All query history is documented for the NHIA's subsequent management purposes. When doctors or hospitals have to download patients' data to integrate it into HIS, they must obtain the patient's written consent before doing so. In addition, the NHIA has established relevant information security management measures to conduct information security inspections on medical institutions that download in batches from time to time.

2. Password Protection

   To further protect personal privacy, doctors and pharmacists will be restricted from querying patients' medical records if those insured set passwords for their NHI IC cards. Setting a password does not affect patients' rights and interests in receiving health care, and medical professionals should provide health care according to the needs of their patients.

Cloud-Based Healthcare Technology Is a Future Trend

Uploading medical information to the NHI MediCloud System enables medical information to be accessed and shared across medical institutions and assists clinical medical professionals in diagnosis and planning patients' follow-up healthcare. Therefore, the concept of "good hospitals in the community; nice doctors in the neighborhood" in the hierarchically integrated medical system policy can be firmed up, and patients' medical care quality and convenience can be improved. Furthermore, the problem of overcrowding in hospitals and overwork of medical professionals can be reduced.

Continuously Upgrading the NHI MediCloud System

The NHI strongly supports and guarantees the social stability and health security of Taiwan. Its wide coverage, easy access, and high quality of care are well-known worldwide. Because of people's expectations of the NHI, the NHIA has innovated and made breakthroughs continuously since its establishment in 1995. The NHI IC card was launched in 2004; in the meantime, the NHI entered a new era of comprehensive informatization. The application of the NHI VPN and centralized information system has enabled contracted medical institutions to fully digitalize claims. With a 93% contracting rate of medical institutions, the National Health Insurance database contains health information of almost all residents in Taiwan, making it a unique national treasure house.

It is convenient for Taiwanese people to seek medical treatment in different hospitals with their NHI IC cards. To allow doctors to review the medications, examinations, and tests uploaded by different medical institutions, the NHIA has established a patient-centered "NHI MediCloud System" for medical institutions to query patients' recent medical records and/or medical images. In addition to linking to websites directly, methods such as batch download and the Application Programming Interface (API) connection have also been launched in response to information development, so that medical institutions can use the in-house information system for data innovation and value-added applications. The achievements were shared in the "Benchmarking Sharing Session on the NHI MediCloud System" on the annual demonstration of this successful public–private partnership. The infrastructure works in line with national policies (so was quickly employed in COVID-19 epidemic prevention in 2020) and establishes a solid foundation on the development of AI.

Applying the Technology to Provide Reminders Proactively

The NHI MediCloud System collects 12 categories of medical information, which is quite diverse and rich. However, medical professionals usually have to make decisions in a split second. By combining information system that provides medical professionals with "information" for clinical practice reference speedily via the HIS, which the medical staff are familiar with, the NHI MediCloud System maximizes the benefits and demonstrates the true value of cloud systems.

Previously, owing to the lack of information circulation, seeking health care in different hospitals often led to duplicated prescriptions or drug interactions, which adversely impacted people's health and caused a waste of resources of the NHI. In addition to providing sufficient information, the NHI MediCloud System shoulders the responsibility of reminding physicians in a more active way to ensure patient safety. Therefore, the NHIA promoted an "Active reminder for duplicated orders" in September 2018 and launched an "Active reminder for drug–drug interactions and/

or allergies" and an "Active reminder of traditional Chinese and Western medicine interaction" in 2019 and 2020 respectively. Innovative technologies were applied to calculate and analyze data actively, and then remind physicians immediately.

The so-called active reminder refers to the quick and instant data exchange between the NHI MediCloud System and the HIS of the medical institutions through the API connection. Before a physician issues a prescription, the information of the prescription is sent to the NHIA through the API, compared with the NHIA big data in real time, and then the physician immediately receives feedback on whether there is a duplication for the current prescription, any interactions with the remaining medicine, or any medicine that patient is allergic to (Fig. 6.5). The connection between the NHI MediCloud System, and the hospital HIS that physicians are accustomed to can be completed within 1–3 s in the same window, which saves physicians time and effort spent on browsing a large quantity of information, as well as enhancing patient safety and medical efficiency.

In addition, medical costs related to kidney disease have remained high in recent years. Kidney function impairment causes patients to enter a course of dialysis, which severely impacts on patients' quality of life. To avoid nonsteroidal anti-inflammatory drugs (NSAIDs), contrast media, and other nephrotoxic drugs from causing further kidney damage to patients with renal dysfunction, the NHIA added "Renal Dysfunction Reminders" in the summary area of the NHI MediCloud System in 2019, and an "Active reminder for NSAID drug usage" in 2020 to remind physicians to review and pay attention to drug prescriptions for specific risk groups.

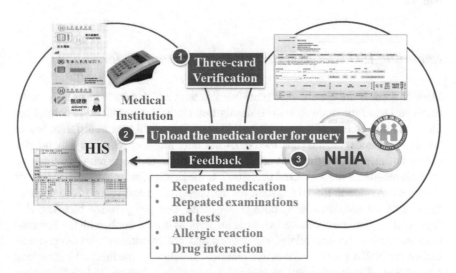

Fig. 6.5 The active reminder function of the NHI MediCloud system

Image Upload, Retrieval, and Sharing

The NHIA started the promotion of medical image-sharing mechanism in 2018 to prevent radiation exposure caused by unnecessary examinations and reduce the waste of medical resources. This mechanism breaks through the limitations of the image retrieval system, formats, and storage space. The NHIA encourages medical institutions to upload imaging data of the patient to the NHI database, so that the doctors from other hospitals can access the images in the NHI MediCloud System through medical image sharing. It reduces patients' cost of transportation, time, and money when applying for video disks from the hospital to seek a second opinion or follow-up care from other hospitals. It also reduces the radiation exposure hazards that the patient may be exposed to when repeatedly undergoing imaging examinations. It is estimated that by sharing CT images and MRI, approximately New Taiwan dollars (NTD) 5.98 million in image reproduction fees and travel time costs were saved every month for the society as a whole.

Medical imaging is an important tool for assisting physicians in diagnosis and disease treatment. In recent years, high-tech imaging examinations such as CT and MRI have been widely used, and their related expenses have always ranked in the top few in the proportions of medical expenses of the NHI. However, repeated medical imaging has the same problem as repeated medications. Physicians may order the examinations owing to professional considerations such as the necessity to check different parts, changes in condition, but it is likely that some examinations are truly unnecessary. It is hoped that through information sharing and decisions made jointly by physicians and patients, in addition to medical necessity, patients must understand the risks of repeated examinations, and cherish medical resources by avoiding unnecessary imaging examinations to achieve the goal of multiparty win-win.

Importing ISO Certification to Protect Personal Information

Medical records are classified as sensitive data with a high degree of privacy in the Personal Data Protection Act. Considering that medical information is helpful for the safety and quality of care when people receive medical care in different hospitals and promotes holistic care, the NHIA not only provides real-time data queries online but also allows the contracted medical institutions to batch download the medical records of the registered patients. The medication, examination, and test are batch downloaded to the HIS system for data integration and value-added applications, such as automatic drug-dosage decisions, and preoperative bleeding risk checks. However, the contracted medical institutions must comply with the Personal Data Protection Act and related regulations and obtain patients' written consent. Before the NHIA provides the active reminder function, some medical institutions have already downloaded patient medical information in batches to build a pop-up reminder in the HIS system to alert doctors. It is especially effective in medication integration, reduction of repeated medications, examinations, and tests of outpatients in hospitals, as well as the prevention of drug interactions.

To ensure that the medical information of the public is fully protected and preserved, the NHIA has set up the "Principles of Batch Download Operation of the NHI MediCloud System for the Contracted Medical Institution" to standardize the implementation of batch download. The institutions should delete the relevant information immediately after completing the consultation (if preservation is necessary, the medical record preservation regulations must be followed). In addition, self-assessment must be conducted every year according to the checklist established by the operation principles. The NHIA will conduct on-site inspections to ensure that the institutes implement the personal data and information security protection.

The Cyber Security Management Act was announced in 2018 and the Regulations on the Classification of Cyber Security Responsibility Levels was amended in 2019 to effectively formulate the cyber security management policies and construct a secure cyber communication environment through the hierarchical management. Taking the agencies with level A cyber security responsibility (such as medical centers) as an example, their core cyber security system should integrate the Chinese National Standards (CNS) 27001/International Organization for Standardization (ISO) 27001 and other Information Security Management System (ISMS) and should be verified by a fair third party. In line with the previous acts and regulations, the NHIA encourages institutions that implement batch downloads to include the NHI MediCloud System batch download operation into the scope of hospital CNS 27001/ISO 27001 certification to standardize management procedures, simplify the trial of batch download, and further ensure the information security protection when utilizing the NHI MediCloud System.

Integrating Information Across Organizations to Safeguard the Health of All Residents

To provide doctors with reference for holistic care, the NHIA not only improves the NHI data integration, but also focuses on cross-organizational information integration. For example, the link to the homepage of the medical institution Electronic Medical Record Exchange Center was added to the examination and test results tab of the NHI MediCloud System in 2017; the NHIA cooperated with the Food and Drug Administration, Ministry of Health and Welfare (MOHW) to promote the report function of the "Drug Therapeutic Inequivalence Reporting System" and establish a drug quality protection mechanism in 2018; the "CDC Vaccinations" tab was added on the NHI MediCloud System at the end of 2018 to provide linkage to the "National Immunization Information System (NIIS)" of the Centers for Disease Control, MOHW; the NHI MediCloud System connects the data of the Taiwan Organ Registry and Sharing Center to provide the function of "comprehensive reporting for overseas organ transplantation" in 2019. The NHIA cooperated with the HPA to import records of adult preventive health care and offer screening results for four major cancers, as well as hepatitis B and hepatitis C, in 2021 to further provide patient-centered diagnosis and treatment.

At the beginning of 2020, the COVID-19 epidemic gradually spread in various countries around the world. The NHIA cooperated with the Central Epidemic Command Center (CECC) to take advantage of the wide use of NHI VPN and the NHI MediCloud System in various medical institutions and quickly integrate the reminder function for travel history of Wuhan and the contact history with confirmed cases provided by the CDC in the NHI MediCloud System. As soon as the patient's NHI IC card is inserted, the system will immediately display a pop-up window to remind the medical institution to pay attention to the patient's condition. Based on the overall epidemic prevention measures, the reminders have been expanded to travel history in various countries, specific high-risk occupations and cluster, referral for further COVID-19 examinations, and whether patients were prescribed with influenza antiviral drugs within 10 days. Through integrating information from the MOHW, National Immigration Agency of the Ministry of the Interior (MOI), the Civil Aeronautics Administration of the Ministry of Transportation and Communications, and the Veterans Affairs Council (Fig. 6.6), the NHI MediCloud System provides medical institutions at all levels (including contracted and noncontracted medical institutions), long-term care institutions, and administrative

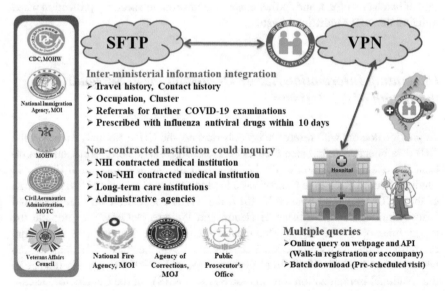

Fig. 6.6 The integrated interministerial information safeguards the national epidemic prevention. SFTP = secure file transfer protocol

agencies (the National Fire Agency of the MOI, the Agency of Corrections of the Ministry of Justice, and the local public prosecutor office) with multiple queries such as online queries (with/without the NHI card), batch download, or API connect, to access epidemic prevention information such as travel history, occupation, contact history, and cluster (TOCC) of incoming and outgoing personnel (Fig. 6.7). The abovementioned information was used to reduce the risk of nosocomial infection and the infection spreading in clusters and communities, reduce internal pressure and infection risks of medical staff and executives, effectively control the spread of diseases, and comprehensively prevent cluster infections. According to statistics, the total number of TOCC inquiries reached nearly 1.18 billion persontimes from February 2020 to September 2021.

The flexible data connection, real-time query, and convenience of the NHI MediCloud System enables it to exert its powerful additional value at this time, so that medical staff can feel more at ease and avoid exposing themselves to danger. Although it is unexpected, the NHI MediCloud System plays an important role in epidemic prevention.

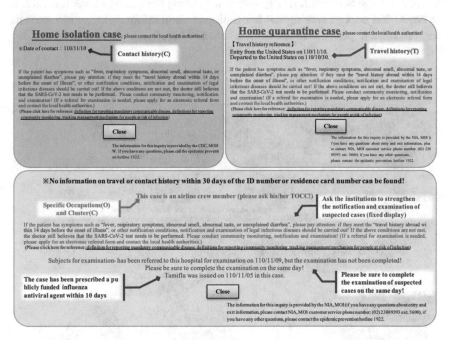

Fig. 6.7 The epidemic prevention information reminder window such as travel history, occupation, contact history, and cluster of the Continuous National Health Insurance MediCloud System upgrade enables smart medical care

Continuous NHI MediCloud System Upgrade Enables Smart Medical Care

The query rate of the NHI MediCloud System has reached nearly 90% since its establishment in 2013. The medical information shared through the NHI MediCloud System and active reminder function significantly reduced the number of unnecessary prescriptions. It is estimated that the cost of repeated drugs reduced by about NTD 9.35 billion from 2014 to 2020, and the cost of repeated examinations and tests was reduced by 1 billion RVUs in 44 categories from 2018 to 2020. Facing the challenges of global population aging, disease treatment, and medical care, it is crucial to promote policies that facilitate innovative application of big data. On the premise of ensuring patient privacy and compliance with relevant laws and regulations, the NHIA will also continuously upgrade the NHI MediCloud System to respond to the development of information and communication technology and the needs of clinical practice (Fig. 6.8). At the same time, it is the ongoing mission of the NHIA to optimize the online query interface of the NHI MediCloud System, provide functions and data with content and interval that are more in line with clinical practice needs to fulfill its key role in improving the quality of medical care. It is hoped that through sharing and integrating medical information, we can exert its highest value to promote smart medical care and benefit the whole population.

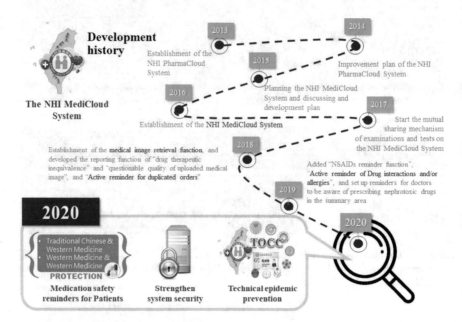

Fig. 6.8 Development history of the National Health Insurance MediCloud System

The National Health Insurance Information Security Management System and Data Protection Mechanism

To abide by the national policy of "Cyber Security is National Security" and to defend increasingly sophisticated cyberattacks, the NHIA improves its information security management mechanism continuously to ensure the security of information systems and national personal data, thereby protecting the information security of the country.

Continuous Improvement of the Information Security Management Mechanism

The NHIA cooperated with the "Implementing a National Information and Communication Infrastructure Security Mechanism Plan" of the National Information and Communication Security Taskforce and imported the ISMS in accordance with the requirements of the "Grading Operations Implementation Plan for Government Agencies' Information Security Responsibility Level." The NHIA owned the domestic and international information security standards obtaining two information security licenses in 2004, and then followed the cyclical improvement spirit of the ISO Plan-Do-Check-Act continuing to promote and strengthen overall cyber security to this day. The NHIA documents and standardizes all information system-relevant operation procedures, including computer room security management, cyber security management, information application system development and management, information access control operations, information security risk assessment and management, business continuity management, and computer virus prevention operations. In addition, the NHIA verifies that the ISMS and information security are in line with domestic and international information security standards through practices such as information asset inventory and risk assessment, internal audit, business continuity plan, management reviews, and on-site audits by impartial third-party auditing agencies. Continuously improving the information security management mechanism through the above methods to ensure the sustainable development of information system operation under the premise of safety and security.

Defense-in-Depth Mechanism Implementation and Internal and External Network Isolation Policies

To ensure the overall information security, the NHIA gradually adjusted the original distributed network architecture to single portal architecture, integrated related information systems into a centralized system architecture, and promoted the construction of dual operation centers in Taipei and Taichung for mutual backup. In addition, firewalls, intrusion detection and defense mechanisms, email filtering, application firewalls, measures against advanced persistent threat, antivirus and antispyware, database accessing and monitoring mechanisms, and intranet firewalls are deployed layer by layer from the external network to the internal network (Fig. 6.9). The NHIA also built a Security Operation Center operating 24 h a day, 365 days a year, and assigned dedicated professional information technology personnel for supervision to prevent intrusion by any malicious threats (Fig. 6.10).

As internet access is the main intrusion channel for any malicious threats, the NHIA has implemented a policy of isolation between the internal and external networks to ensure the overall security of the internal network. Colleagues can only connect to the internet through the external Virtual Desktop Infrastructure mechanism to block possible internet threats from the external network (Fig. 6.11).

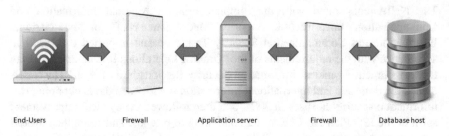

Fig. 6.9 Defense-in-depth mechanism

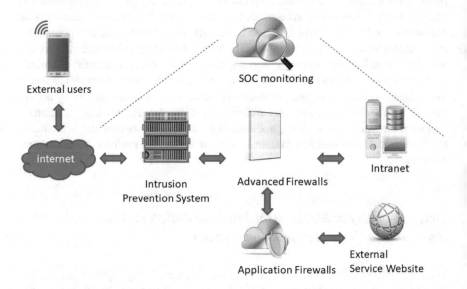

Fig. 6.10 External service protection mechanism

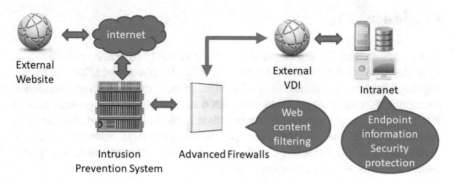

Fig. 6.11 Intranet protection mechanism

Regular Information Security Testing and Drills to Reduce the Potential Risks of Information Security

The NHIA is a government agency compliant with information security responsibility level A, which regularly conducts two website security vulnerability detections and repairs, one penetration test that simulates hacking techniques, and one information security inspection annually. We hope to find out and fix the potential risks of the information system architecture through regular self-review to avoid being used by hackers. The NHIA also implemented the most advanced Red Team Assessment attack in 2018. Under the premise of not affecting the operation of the NHIA, the practice conducts simulated intrusion attacks on the organization, executes attacks from various entry points in a limited time in an all-purpose way, tries to achieve the test tasks designated by the NHIA, as well as exploring potential risks and fixing them.

Implement Database ID Entity Encryption Mechanism

The large amount of highly sensitive medical claim data from contracted institutions collected by the NHIA is coveted by all parties (computer hackers, data brokers, fraudulent groups, etc.), and it is always facing the threat of intrusion and stealing by interested parties in various ways. In view of the foregoing circumstances, the NHIA conducted related research on data encryption in 2008, and the results showed that only a small number of operations may need to display plaintext data. Subsequently, the medical data transferred from the external to the NHIA will be encrypted (Database ID entity encryption mechanism), and the relevant information system will be fully renovated to ensure that the information and business personnel cannot have contact with the true plaintext data during the business process and reduce the possibility of data leakage. In addition, the underwriting database of the NHI was also implemented in 2013; the data provided by the Data Warehouse to external agency passes two encryption operations to ensure the security of people's personal data.

Conclusion

Taiwan has entered the era of value-added use of medical, health, and care data. With the promotion of a smart health policy by the government, the NHIA has improved the quality and efficiency of medical services by introducing information communication technology. Combined with data analysis and a high transmission rate through 5G applications, the design and promotion of the virtual NHI card will continue to be in line with the vision of fostering open application and industrial development, so that the public can obtain medical services more conveniently with more choices as we start a new era of care.

Chapter 7
Innovative Applications of the Medical Information

Po-Chang Lee, Shwu-Huey Wu, Yu-Pin Chang, and Joyce Tsung-Hsi Wang

Introduction

Telemedicine has become a useful tool for delivering health care to patients in remote areas or COVID-19 patients in quarantine. There are two ways of providing telemedicine under current regulations. Teleconsultations between doctors, especially for seeking second opinions from different specialists or patients can obtain medical diagnosis, and treatment made through telecommunications directly when they are under quarantine. Patients can receive proper medical care without the restriction of distance, and the risk of disease transmission can also be minimized. The application of 5G technology further creates a better environment for healthcare delivery. Using the virtual National Health Insurance (NHI) card displayed on a mobile device to support telemedicine and home-based medical care is the best example of providing comprehensive health care by combining information and communication technology (ICT) and health care in the digital healthcare era.

During the COVID-19 pandemic, the National Health Insurance MediCloud System (NHI MediCloud System) provided travel history, occupation, contact history, and cluster (TOCC) to medical providers for epidemic control, and the NHI VPN system was used to distribute masks through the contracted pharmacies in the early stage of the epidemic. Although the application of the NHI database is increasing, the issue of secondary use of NHI data is a concern. Therefore, the balance between innovations and securing people's rights and privacy needs further discussion to find an appropriate way to use the NHI data.

P.-C. Lee (✉) · S.-H. Wu · Y.-P. Chang · J. T.-H. Wang
National Health Insurance Administration, Ministry of Health and Welfare, Taipei, Taiwan
e-mail: pochang@nhi.gov.tw; shwu@nhi.gov.tw; A110413@nhi.gov.tw; mdjoyce@nhi.gov.tw

The Important Milestone: "2021—First Year of Telemedicine Being Covered"

In view of the arrival of the Internet era, the advances in technology products, and the demands of the aging society, the Ministry of Health and Welfare (MOHW) issued the "Rules of Medical Diagnosis and Treatment by Telecommunications" on 11 May 2018. The rules liberalize those insured who are eligible to receive telemedicine and constitute a scheme under which telemedicine could be delivered. Besides mountainous areas, outlying islands, remote areas, and urgent circumstances, the patients could also receive diagnosis and treatment by electronic ICT under the following five special circumstances.

1. Acute inpatients who require follow-up treatment within 3 months after being discharged.
2. Residents of long-term care institutions who require diagnosis or treatment by the physicians because of their medical conditions.
3. Patients who are specified under relevant laws and regulations to be in need of integrated care require diagnosis or treatment by family physicians because of their medical conditions.
4. The telecare programs approved by competent authorities, or follow-up treatment for patients with home-based medical care within 3 months after diagnosis and treatment from the physicians.
5. Foreign patients who are without citizenship and absent from the NHI.

After the laws and regulations were expanded, the National Health Insurance Administration (NHIA) began a pilot telemedicine program to provide telemedicine services for people in remote areas.

The COVID-19 Pandemic Accelerates the Inclusion of Telemedicine into the Benefits Package of the National Health Insurance

In response to the need for diagnosis and treatment through telecommunications due to the impact of the COVID-19 epidemic, the MOHW expanded the insured eligibility of telemedicine in February 2020 to people with medical needs when they are in home quarantine, home isolation, and self-management of health. The expenses of the diagnosis and treatment through telecommunications are covered by the NHI when the patients are people who are complying with isolation and quarantine regulation and who have been referred by the local health authority because of urgent medical needs other than fever or respiratory symptoms.

As the epidemic ravaged and impacted the healthcare system, medical institutions and the public realized the necessity of telemedicine, which facilitated the inclusion of telemedicine in the benefits of the NHI.

Inclusion of Telemedicine in the Fee Schedule in 2021

Teleconsultation between doctors provides diversified medical channels for people in remote areas, which enhances medical accessibility and optimizes utilization of medical resources. Specialists from afar are brought to the public through medical technology to conduct medical consultation effectively. This realizes the goal of providing medical care and treatment in place, whereas patients are able to receive the health care they need without traveling. For cases that cannot be treated remotely, the referral service would be arranged immediately to effectively seize the golden period of treatment.

The top priority of the "National Health Insurance Telemedicine Coverage Plan" implemented in 2021 was to promote the cooperation between medical institutions in mountainous areas, outlying islands, and remote areas and those with more medical resources. Local physicians in mountainous areas, outlying islands, and remote areas are now able to examine patients in person while specialists in remote sites (which can be doctors in medical centers, regional hospitals, district hospitals, and clinics) examine patients through ICT and provide advice. Special medical care (ophthalmology, otolaryngology, dermatology) or emergency treatments that are lacking in the local area and urgently needed will be the main focus in the early stage of implementation. By providing teleconsultation services, specialists receive 500 relative value units (RVUs) per person or 5000 RVUs per visit. As for the emergency teleconsultation, it is paid according to its level of triage classification, ranging from 507 to 2340 RVUs per person per visit.

Digital Technology Extends Medical Care

Teleconsultation in Taiwan refers to local doctors and online doctors discussing the patient's condition together. The patient's notations on the NHI card and medical information (such as the medication information in the "NHI MediCloud System") must be available to the physician providing a remote consultation as background information. In response to the trend of mobile smart health, the new generation of the NHI card is designed as a virtual NHI card, and pilots will be conducted in the fields of "home-based medical care" and "teleconsultation" (applying 5G) to fill service gaps in the current healthcare system. The public will be able to authenticate and build a personal virtual NHI card through the "National Health Insurance Mobile Easy Access mobile application (NHI Express app)." It is expected that in the future, medical personnel who execute teleconsultation will be able to access the NHI's data (such as images, medicines, and medical records) by reading virtual NHI cards, and provide medical services to people in remote areas.

Inconvenient transportation is the main cause of time and cost waste for the elderly population or people with impaired mobility in remote areas when seeking medical care in public health centers or other hospitals and clinics. After taking issues such as home network bandwidth, information security, patient privacy, and mobile device availability into consideration, the needs to deliver teleconsultation or telecare into patients' home still exist. Therefore, it is our goal to provide patients with teleconsultation in their homes through ICT (for example: the virtual NHI card, the NHI MediCloud System) in the future.

Telemedicine breaks through the limitation of distance so that medical resources can be utilized in a more efficient manner. We are in the process of introducing telemedicine into the NHI Fee Schedule and Reference List for Medical Service, so that it can be provided by medical institutions as a regular service item. By providing physicians in the clinics with consultation with specialist doctors from major hospitals, we can make better use of the referral system and construct a telemedicine payment system that meets our needs. Coupled with the development of digital technology, we look forward to further extending our service to telecare and combine medical and long-term care together.

The Major Stride of Health Insurance Information Network and Far-Reaching Medical Services Made Possible by 5G

Brief Talk About the Health Insurance Information Network

The comprehensive replacement of the NHI paper card with the NHI IC card in 2004 is an important milestone. To provide a smoother connection when accessing patient information with the NHI card and safer data transmission, the NHIA also commissioned Chunghwa Telecom to construct a brand-new National Health Insurance Virtual Private Network (hereinafter referred to as the NHI VPN). Features of VPN are:

1. Because the information systems that transfer relatively confidential and sensitive information or transaction content, such as financial institution transactions (automatic teller machine, ATM), credit card swiping and receipt operations, and the lottery coupon endorsement station system all adopt private network architecture and transmission mode, the NHI VPN is also built as a private network.
2. Only contracted medical institutions and medical information vendors approved by the NHIA can join the NHI VPN. Therefore, it is easy to identify a user's identity and manage, greatly reducing hacker intrusion. This feature makes it easier to detect the source when a virus attack or network abnormality occurs and ensures health insurance data transmission security.
3. The network infrastructure and management are equal to enterprise-level networks. Hence, its connection speed, packet effectiveness, and bandwidth priority are better than those of the general Internet, effectively ensuring smooth operation.

4. There is no location restriction. Whether the contracted medical institution is located in the city, remote island, or mountainous area, it is charged at the same price and provides the same network service level.
5. Originally, the VPN only supported NHI IC card connection operation and claims submission; then, it has been expanded to all medical services provided by the NHIA in recent years, such as providers' online data modification, cloud query system for medical information, and image data (referred to as the NHI MediCloud System), and related TOCC information needed in response to the epidemic.

To serve areas where physical network routes are difficult to install, and in response to the advancement of telecommunications technology, the VPN is also continuously expanding from providing a 3G mobile connection to progressing to the current 4G mobile connection.

Enter the 5G Era

With the official launch of 5G in Taiwan in 2020, telecommunications companies and various industries have begun to launch various 5G value-added application services. The VPN gradually upgraded to a 5G mobile connection from 2021 region by region, enabling the healthcare field to deliver more application services.

Compared with the current 4G, 5G technology has the advantages of high speed and low latency, so that the time spent on transferring large amounts of data and medical images is greatly reduced, helping to improve the timeliness of NHI VPN services.

Convenient medical services that the NHIA currently provides or expects to implement with 5G technology are:

1. Teleconsultation between doctors

   (a) To improve the quality and efficiency of medical care in rural areas, enrich local medical resources, and implement healthcare localization, the MOHW announced "The Rules of Medical Diagnosis and Treatment by Telecommunications." In 2021, the NHIA launched a pilot program that covers teleconsultation between doctors provided in mountainous areas and outlying islands (50 towns) across the country and areas designated by the MOHW.

   (b) Through the assistance of the information system, the treatment, diagnosis service, and consultation for a patient in this plan are provided by remote specialist doctors (medical center or large hospital site) and the local doctor (patient site) jointly. The local doctor then prescribes medical orders for specialist doctors' follow-up.

   (c) The local physician is equipped with specific medical equipment, such as ophthalmoscopes, to transfer real-time, high-resolution medical images or video data through 5G technology. In this way, the remote specialist doctors could treat and diagnose as if the patient is in front of them and provide immediate feedback to the local physician, providing the patient with a complete illness description and professional advice.

2. Home-based medical care

    (a) Home-based medical care refers to dispatching a team of medical providers from a contracted hospital to the home of the people who have signed up for home-based medical care. The most obvious advantage of home-based medical care is to improve the medical care accessibility of patients with mobility impairments and reduce the inconvenience and time cost of going out in person.

    (b) The NHIA has many years of experience in promoting this service. Initially, the target audience is those people with mobility impairments, and it was subsequently expanded to patients with chronic mental illness and hospice patients, respirator-dependent patients. Home-based medical care was also provided to support nursing institutions and nursing homes. A complete home-based medical care integration platform has been established under the "NHIA Home-Based Medical Care Integration Plan."

    (c) To alleviate the home-based medical care teams' burden of carrying NHI IC card-customized readers, a pilot trial program was conducted in the central region of Taiwan in 2018 to replace laptops/computers with mobile phones. After reviewing and improving the pilot program's effectiveness, the "Home-Based Medical Care Bluetooth Lightweight Project" was launched, so that home-based medical care teams no longer need to carry bulky laptops/computers, customized card readers, and uninterruptible power supply equipment, etc. Instead, by operating the Home-Based Medical Care app developed by the NHIA installed on a mobile phone and a handy Bluetooth card reader, medical providers can still access patients' health information by reading their NHI IC cards.

    (d) At present, mobile phones only connect to the VPN through 4G technology. Soon, 5G will be adopted for faster and more convenience when querying cloud data, even pictures and medical images, etc. It also makes real-time interactive discussion with hospital professionals possible, providing home-based medical care patients with better professional care.

Future Direction

The NHIA is working on contingency measures to tackle issues derived from the COVID-19 pandemic. For example, when people under quarantine need medical attention, remote doctors can diagnose and prescribe through the 5G Internet connection without exposing them to the risk of contact infection (Fig. 7.1). The NHIA will continue to improve the current two-way data exchange between the "Integrated Home-Based Medical Care Platform System" and other MOHW systems (such as

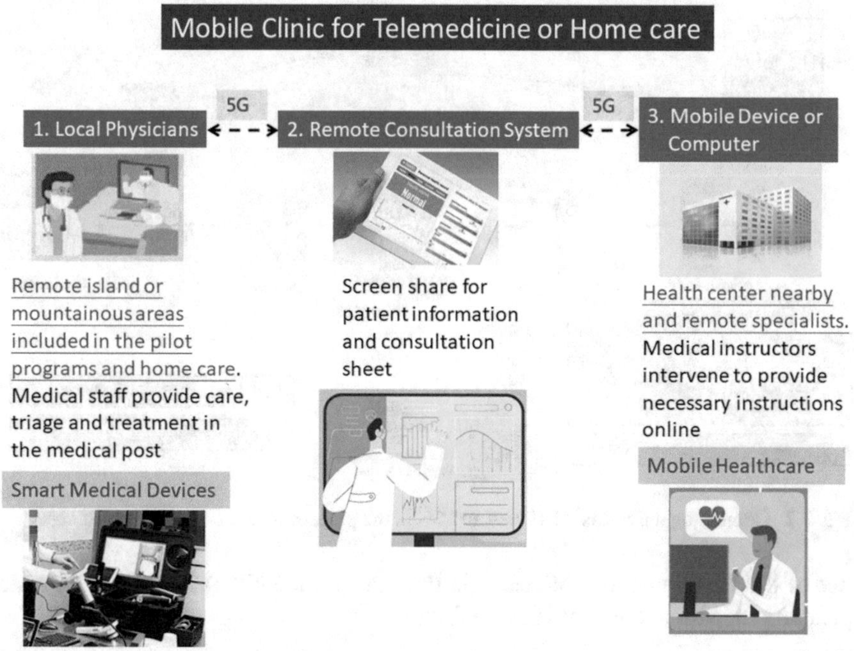

Fig. 7.1 Workflow of online medical consultation via 5G internet in telemedicine and home-based medical care

long-term care management systems) to reduce users' redundant data entry, to overcome the inconvenience of cross-platform referrals and case receptions, making the home-based medical care delivery process smoother. It is hoped that home-based medical care teams' workload on data processing when returning to the hospital after a day out can be reduced. Combined with the virtual NHI card pilot program launched in 2020, we look forward to developing a better practice model in the future (Fig. 7.2).

With the assistance of 5G technology and continuous efforts, the NHIA is more confident in fulfilling the promise of providing comprehensive healthcare to all citizens in each township.

Virtual NHI Card Users in the 5G Era

In Taiwan, as long as you hold a valid NHI card, you can go to nearly 30,000 NHI contracted medical institutions to receive different types of medical services, including Western medicine, traditional Chinese medicine, and dental care, according to your own health needs. People may receive high-quality outpatient care, inpatient care, surgery, medical tests, and medications. During the COVID-19 epidemic, the utilization of the NHI card for TOCC reminders and name-based mask purchase was tremendously crucial. However, when people had taken to the current NHI card as

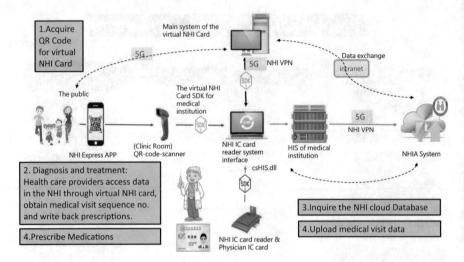

Fig. 7.2 Combining the virtual NHI card and 5G in the process of home-based medical care

one of the most indispensable cards in their purses, the NHIA had already started planning the virtual NHI card for the future.

Planning for a New Generation NHI Card

The NHIA had completely replaced the previously paper card with the NHI IC card in 2004, which was widely recognized in all walks of life (Fig. 7.3). However, it has been more than 17 years since then. To echo the "Mobile Payments" promoted by the Executive Yuan and meet the demands of mobile smart health, the reform of the NHI card is carried out with a forward-looking perspective to fit the vision of the Digital Nation and Innovative Economic Development Program. Therefore, the NHIA cooperated with the Public Digital Innovation Space of the Executive Yuan to invite the public, physicians, pharmacists, nurses, public associations, experts, and scholars to hold three collaborative meetings on 4 July, 8 August, and 26 November 2018, to gather opinions from all parties (Fig. 7.4). In these collaborative meetings, these stakeholders concluded that the planning of the new-generation NHI cards will not contain biometric information, and the principles are set as follows:

1. Virtual and physical cards will be used simultaneously. Retain the current physical NHI card system and gradually develop virtual NHI cards.
2. Pilot project: the virtual NHI card will be used on a trial basis and will be fully implemented after the testing is completed.
3. Mainly for medical care: the NHI card is for medical use and will not include other add-on functions, such as electronic payment.

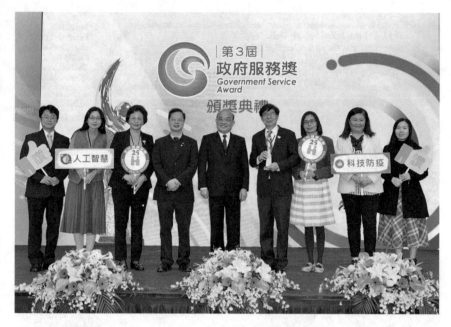

Fig. 7.3 In December 2020, the NHIA won the "Digital Innovation Value-Added Prize" in the competition of the 3rd Government Service Award. Premier Su Tseng-Chang presented the award to NHIA Director General Lee. (From Executive Yuan. https://www.ey.gov.tw/Page/9277F759E41CCD91/b7b9672b-f581-4d04-bc3f-2c68ee54d2e3)

The Virtual NHI Card Pilot Program

The NHIA has developed a medical service model for the virtual NHI card on a trial basis since 2018. People can download the NHI Express app on their mobile phones and apply for a virtual NHI card. When seeking medical care, instead of handing in the physical IC cards to providers, patients can display the virtual NHI card's QR code to the medical institution for scanning (Fig. 7.5). In addition, when medical professionals need to access the NHI MediCloud System to obtain patients' medication records and examination reports, they can scan the virtual NHI card's QR code for authentication along with the medical institution card and physician card, to enhance medication safety and facilitate medical treatment (Fig. 7.6).

Comments and experience of different levels of medical institutions, pharmacies, rehabilitation and treatment institutions, and home-based medical care were collected to understand their obstacles, difficulties, and impact while using virtual NHI cards. Opinions of different stakeholders such as people seeking medical care, medical service providers, and medical information system providers were also collected before the NHIA evaluates the feasibility, advantages and disadvantages, information security, and personal information protection of the virtual NHI card and conducted a cost analysis.

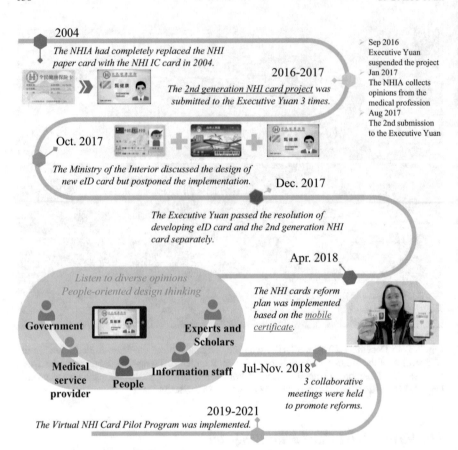

Fig. 7.4 The history of the virtual NHI card. (The portrait of Audrey Tang is licensed by Audrey Tang. Source: https://www.cw.com.tw/article/5109960)

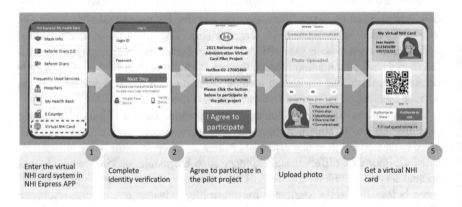

Fig. 7.5 How to display the virtual National Health Insurance (NHI) card on smart phones by verifying identity on the NHI Express app

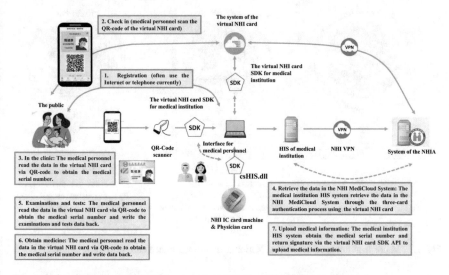

Fig. 7.6 The flow of medical visits using virtual National Health Insurance card

The result of the trial shows that 83% of people want to apply for a virtual NHI card; 93% of the people who received home-based medical care would like to use virtual NHI cards to obtain drugs of refillable chronic illness prescriptions, and 94% of them suggest increasing the function of dependents.

The virtualization of the NHI card substantially improves the accessibility to medical treatment such as home-based medical care and telemedicine for people who reside in remote areas and offshore islands and those with impaired mobility. It also relieves medical practitioners from the burden of carrying multiple heavy pieces of equipment when doing home visits. Furthermore, for people receiving home-based medical care or telemedicine, the caregivers who escort them to visit and obtain medication for them are often different people, making passing the NHI card around very inconvenient. This can be easily avoided by using the dependents function of the virtual NHI card. Therefore, the pilot participants highly support obtaining home-based medical care and telemedicine with the virtual NHI cards.

Continuous Function Progresses

It is our goal to expand the use of the virtual NHI card to fields such as home-based medical care and telemedicine, which have higher benefits than their costs and unmet needs that current medical information services cannot provide. The main focus of the virtual NHI card pilot program in 2021 is to provide medical services to settings where the current delivery system fails to meet the needs of the public, including 'home-based medical care' and 'teleconsultations,' to address the

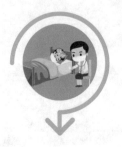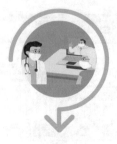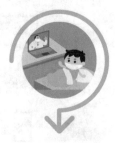

Home-based Medical Care

- Alleviate the burden of equipment doctors and nurses have to carry
- Reduced the inconvenience of family members

Teleconsultations for Rural areas

- Doctors on both sides can access the information of patients by scanning the QR Code of the virtual NHI card

Telemedicine for the quarantined and more

- People can get medical care by using virtual card without going to the hospitals to complete the process.

Fig. 7.7 Major trial fields of the virtual National Health Insurance card pilot program in 2021

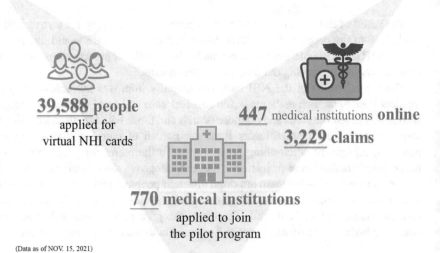

39,588 people
applied for
virtual NHI cards

447 medical institutions **online**
3,229 claims

770 **medical institutions**
applied to join
the pilot program

(Data as of NOV. 15, 2021)

Fig. 7.8 The outcome of the virtual National Health Insurance card pilot program in 2021

problem of medical accessibility (Fig. 7.7). Now, more than 440 medical institutions have completed the installation of the virtual NHI card system (Fig. 7.8). By closing the current service gap, reducing the equipment medical practitioners need to carry, improving the efficiency of medical services, we look forward to enhancing the convenience, fairness, and satisfaction of people seeking medical care to

Home care and telemedicine fields

We are going to fill gap of the current medical system and satisfy the needs of the NHI medical services from the perspective of the general public.

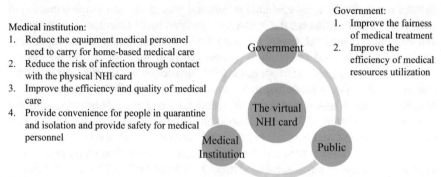

Medical institution:
1. Reduce the equipment medical personnel need to carry for home-based medical care
2. Reduce the risk of infection through contact with the physical NHI card
3. Improve the efficiency and quality of medical care
4. Provide convenience for people in quarantine and isolation and provide safety for medical personnel

Government:
1. Improve the fairness of medical treatment
2. Improve the efficiency of medical resources utilization

Public:
1. Improve the convenience of seeking medical care for patients with chronic diseases
2. Improve the convenience of home-based medical care, medical care for people with impaired mobility, and medicine obtainment for caregivers
3. Improve the efficiency of medical resource utilization
4. Provide convenience for people in quarantine and isolation and provide safety for medical personnel

Fig. 7.9 The virtual National Health Insurance card is used in home-based medical care and telemedicine fields to create win-win-win benefits

maximize benefits and create an all-win situation for the government, medical institutions, and the people (Fig. 7.9).

Using the National Health Insurance Information System for COVID-19 Prevention

Since the NHIA launched the NHI MediCloud System in 2013, it has stably provided 24-h nonstop inter-hospital medical information inquiry service. At the beginning of 2020, owing to the outbreak of COVID-19 in China, the Central Epidemic Command Center (CECC) assigned the NHIA to integrate the cross-departmental data. The NHIA has built a travel history and contact history reminder function to fully support medical institutions in preventing the spread of COVID-19 and avoiding the risk of infection for frontline medical staff. Although it was the Chinese lunar New Year holiday at that time, owing to the urgency and timeliness of the epidemic, the NHIA still urgently mobilized manpower and third-party vendors. First, manually perform data clean-up and import it into the NHI cloud database. At the same time, the first version of the TOCC reminder function implementation was completed highly efficiently within 2 days. It was officially launched on 27 January 2020 (the third day of the lunar New Year) for inquiries by contracted medical institutions.

The Cross-Departmental Cooperation of the National Health Insurance Cloud System to Add a TOCC Reminder

In response to the different epidemic prevention procedures and usage scenarios of various medical institutions, the NHIA later enabled batch downloads, web service and other data connect channels, provided medical institutions with the rapid integration of the Hospital Information System (HIS) to improve the overall convenience of epidemic prevention operations. We also continued to refine the reminder function of the system according to the instructions of the CECC. For example, in March 2020, the NHIA added high-risk occupations and cluster history, referral for examination, and other reminders, to cooperate with the "Strengthening the Infection Control of Medical and Nursing Institutions," and made rolling adjustments based on the epidemic development and the feedback from the medical community (such as priority, number of days, warning text, etc.). Refer to Table 7.1 for a brief description of the key prevention strategies implemented during the pandemic.

Because travel history and other pandemic prevention data are sensitive personal data, to protect information security and prevent the epidemic at the same time, the data exchange between the NHIA and various departments is transmitted through a secure file transfer protocol. Furthermore, the NHIA has developed a more flexible and automated software program to establish a mechanism for data collection, verification and error feedback and improve the accuracy and timeliness of data. The query track of relevant pandemic prevention information is fully encrypted and

Table 7.1 The key prevention strategies implemented through the National Health Insurance (NHI) MediCloud system during the COVID-19 pandemic

Schedule	Execution
January to February 2020	1. In the first version of the system, physicians and pharmacists inquire about travel history and contact history through the patient's NHI card. Later, the NHIA provides the hospitals' self-authorized personnel for inquiring, and those situations such as out-of-pocket medical service or person with no nationality can inquire without an NHI card. In addition, the batch download and Web Service connection channels were provided 2. In the initial stage, only travel information in China, Hong Kong, and Macao areas such as Wuhan City and Hubei Province was presented. Later, according to the instructions, it was gradually expanded to include entry (exit) information for all locations
March 2020	1. Travel and contact history reminder information, which presents at the highest level, is in accordance with the risk of infection. 2. The high-risk occupations, cluster history information, referral for examination, instructions, and reference documents for a notification examination were added
April to May 2020	1. The home isolation (quarantine) cases were suggested to conduct an additional 7-day self-health management after the 14-day isolation (quarantine) 2. In response to telemedicine during the epidemic, the "Inquiry Operations Responding to Natural Disasters and Emergency Medical" was opened, and physicians could inquire about inter-hospital medical information with patient's ID numbers

NHIA National Health Insurance Administration

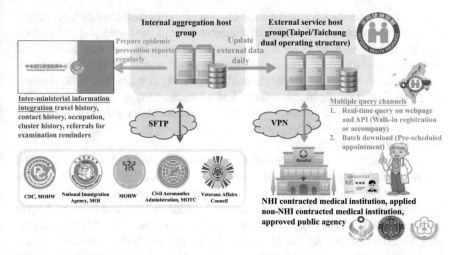

Fig. 7.10 Data exchange and transmission of the "National Health Insurance MediCloud System"

stored in the database of the NHI. The storage and protection of various data are also handled at the highest level of security of the NHIA, and data-cleaning operations are carried out regularly in accordance with regulations. For the data exchange and transmission during this pandemic prevention period, please refer to Fig. 7.10.

One year after the COVID-19 outbreak, in January 2021, the physicians of the Taoyuan General Hospital of the MOHW were diagnosed with infection because they treated imported cases, and their contacts such as related medical staff were also diagnosed with infections. To this end, the CECC announced the launch of the "Project of the Taoyuan General Hospital of the Ministry of Health and Welfare." The NHIA rapidly noted the discharged patients from the hospital, the patients who had been in the hospital's outpatient and emergency department, and the hospital staff. At the beginning of February of the same year, the notes were deleted by the end of the project. Thus, the system once again efficiently and successfully cooperated with the CECC's epidemic prevention work.

Establish a Control System for Masks and Distribute Protective Materials Fairly

It is worth mentioning that in the early stage of the outbreak of the COVID-19 pandemic, medical masks were in surge demand. To make the distribution fair and so that everyone could buy masks smoothly, the Executive Yuan decided to adopt the "name-based mask distribution system" on 3 February 2020. The NHIA deployed its manpower and equipment resources and established the first version of the "name-based mask distribution system" within 3 days as a distribution platform on the NHI VPN environment that each contracted pharmacy was familiar with. People needed to prove their identity with their NHI card when purchasing masks (such as whether they meet the interval days and number of masks they can purchase; people whose card cannot be read, who hold residence permits, and entry and exit permits without an NHI card, can also log in manually by entering their card number and birthday). The name-based mask distribution system was officially launched on 6 February 2020 as scheduled. People could buy masks at more than 6000 pharmacies, 340 district public health centers, and 12 health centers across Taiwan. This distributed people with the suffix of their ID card numbers, greatly reducing the crowds in the line, dispersing system traffic, and solving the chaos of rushing to buy masks in one fell swoop.

In addition, to prevent the people from rushing for masks, the NHIA has been synchronizing the centralized database of the "name-based medical mask distribution system 1.0," such as the detailed list of the remaining number of masks in NHI-contracted institutions and the service hours of the institutions, and released them to the government's open data platform since 6 February. The NHIA has also cooperated with the civil society led by Audrey Tang, Minister without Portfolio of the Executive Yuan to build a "Mask Supply and Demand Information Platform" for public inquiries, and for the private sector and the industry to develop multiple value-added applications. This not only disperses the query traffic on the official website of the NHIA, but also makes the mask system service stable and uninterrupted. The public can easily check the location, inventory, and business hours for purchasing masks in various regions effectively preventing the spread of the domestic epidemic.

Some people reflect that it was difficult to buy masks owing to work or distance to the physical stores. To improve the distribution efficiency and utilization of masks, Minister Tang proposed using digital services and launch the "name-based medical mask distribution system 2.0" so that the public can obtain masks through "preorder online and pick-up at a convenience store." The NHIA immediately invited representatives of Minister Tang, Trade-Van Information Service, and the four major convenience stores to conduct intensive discussions about the online preorder process and system interface operations between departments. Online preorder of masks was officially launched on 12 March 2020. Afterward, the "3.0 Convenience Store Preorder" service was launched, allowing people to pick up the masks they have ordered and preorder more masks at neighboring convenient stores, making it more convenient to obtain masks.

In addition to physical channels and online preorders and refills, the CECC passed a resolution on 17 March 2020 that domestic or international travelers could purchase masks at airport duty-free shops after entering the country. The quantity they purchased were registered in the name-based mask distribution system on the website of the MOHW too. In late March, for high-risk groups for whom it was inconvenient to go out or buy masks online, it was agreed that each responsible unit would distribute masks to the people in the unit. Refer to Fig. 7.11 for the integration of multiple mask purchase channels in the name-based mask distribution system.

The NHIA developed the TOCC and name-based mask distribution system quickly and effectively to assist in epidemic prevention work, using IT systems to help fight COVID-19, arousing the interest of other countries. We are happy to share our successful experience with the world (Figs. 7.12 and 7.13).

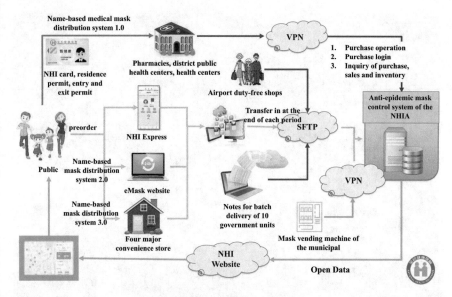

Fig. 7.11 Integration of multiple channels of the "name-based mask distribution system"

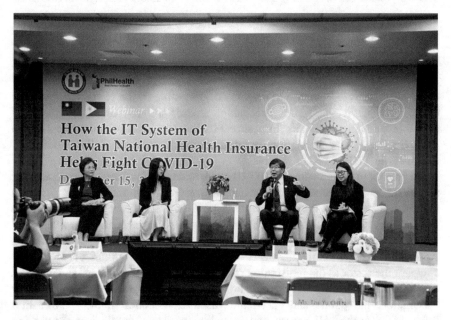

Fig. 7.12 In December 2020, the National Health Insurance Administration held a webinar with PhilHealth on how the IT system of Taiwan National Health Insurance helps to fight COVID-19

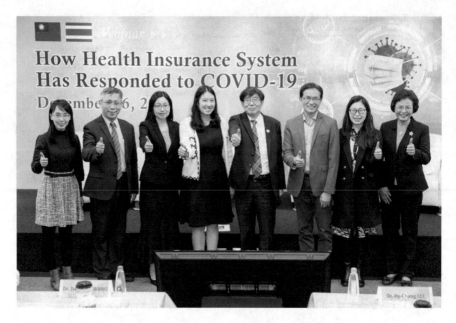

Fig. 7.13 In December 2020, the National Health Insurance Administration held a webinar with Thailand's National Health Security Office on how health insurance has responded to COVID-19

Enhance NHI Express APP and My Health Bank Functions for COVID-19 Prevention [1]

Since May 2021, in response to the COVID-19 outbreak, the NHIA has launched three digital services including vaccination records and test results of COVID-19 available on National Health Insurance Mobile Easy Access mobile application (NHI Express app), deregulation for telemedicine during the COVID-19 outbreak, and the virtual NHI Card Pilot Project.

To prevent infection with COVID-19, more and more institutions have asked for a COVID-19 negative report or vaccination record as an entrance pass. Such a request has become a trend. In response to the CECC's announcement that the COVID-19 vaccine was administered on 22 March 2021, the NHIA also cooperated with the provision of the "COVID-19 Vaccine Registration list Comparison Application Programming Interface." The responsible institutions could quickly compare the roster at the registration counter, follow the professional judgment of the physician and other vaccine situations for reference before vaccination. After vaccination, the public can check the vaccination record in the "Vaccination Information" in the NHI Express app, including the date of vaccination, the vaccine manufacturer, and the place of vaccination. In addition, the NHIA has consolidated COVID-19 vaccination records and records for rapid antigen tests, polymerase chain reaction tests, and antibody tests into My Health Bank system on the NHI Express app as the service named "Vaccination Records and Test Results of

COVID-19." While the CECC is preparing for vaccine passports that are internationally accepted, people in Taiwan can just log into the NHI Express app on their smartphone to present these records anytime and anywhere. It is expected that this service will be widely used in the near future.

In coordination with five major Taiwanese telecommunication companies, since May 2018, the NHIA has used individual cell phone numbers for identity authentication together with their NHI card number to bind their identity to the NHI Express app. With such a convenient approach, people can easily access their COVID-19 vaccination records and test results from their personal My Health Bank account (Fig. 7.14).

Meanwhile, during this pandemic, diagnosis and treatment through telecommunications have greatly helped patients with chronic conditions. For those who need to see a doctor regularly including first-time ambulatory patients and stable chronically ill patients, the NHI can cover them for the use of telemedicine. Therefore, it is also expected that telemedicine will play a more advanced role in the post-epidemic era.

In addition, to facilitate home healthcare and medical services in remote areas, the virtual NHI Card Pilot Project has been launched. This Project in 2021 was aimed at three types of service provided by the NHIA. For home healthcare and medical services in remote areas, a virtual NHI card eases the burden of equipment and also allows the NHI MediCloud System to be reached to gain a patient's further information. When diagnosing and treating patients who are in quarantine with telecommunications, with this virtual NHI card, providers' risk of being infected during subsequent medication dispensing and other administrative procedures is reduced.

Three NHI digital services have been well implemented. Digital technologies applied to healthcare can enhance the health of people and more services will be applied in the future.

NHIA's Role in Information Management

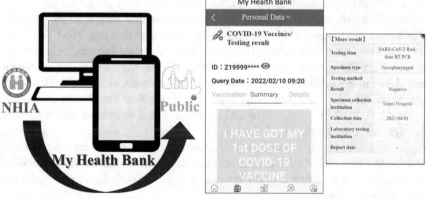

Fig. 7.14 The role of the National Health Insurance Administration in information management

The Name-Based Medical Mask Distribution System Is a Successful Model Established by Government and Private Sector Partnerships to Fight the COVID-19 Pandemic [2]

Owing to the outbreak of COVID-19 in early 2020, Taiwanese people rushed to buy medical masks, causing mask chaos. To make the public feel at ease and ensure a fair opportunity for everyone to buy masks, the government implemented the name-based medical mask distribution system on 6 February 2020. The system enables the public to purchase masks with their NHI cards at contracted pharmacies and health centers across the country.

The name-based medical mask distribution system is a cross-ministerial and cross-organizational cooperation platform on which people can locate the remaining masks in a certain area in real time. The NHIA also releases open datasets such as the mask inventory and information at contracted pharmacies and health centers. The private sectors used the NHI open datasets to develop more than 140 mask map applications that were integrated into the Mask Supply and Demand Information Platform for public use.

This mechanism solved the problem of finding a place to buy face masks and improved the availability of epidemic prevention materials. The NHIA collects opinions from all parties to continuously optimize the system. Later on, the NHIA followed the government policies to facilitate a preorder system online and in convenience stores. Coupled with citizen's compliance with epidemic prevention guidelines, Taiwan's COVID-19 prevention achievement is widely recognized around the world.

Medical Masks Become Popular Anti-epidemic Materials

At the end of 2019, the COVID-19 epidemic was reported in Wuhan and Hubei in China. Wuhan completely stopped public transportation at 10 am on 23 January 2020, indicating that the epidemic had been expanding continuously. Taiwan's CECC elevated the epidemic to the second level on the same day. The CECC worried that the virus would enter Taiwan along with returning Taiwanese citizens and tourists from China, so it instructed the NHIA to display the travel history of Wuhan and Hubei in the system for physicians' reference as soon as possible. The NHIA completed the mission in just 2 days even in the lunar New Year holiday.

As the COVID-19 pandemic spread rapidly, the first confirmed case was found through boarding quarantine before the lunar New Year, and sporadic imported cases were subsequently confirmed. Although the government urgently released medical masks reserved for emergencies to convenience stores, many people rushed to a number of convenience stores but got nothing, which indirectly caused panic about the epidemic.

To consider the effectiveness of epidemic prevention and increase the coverage of masks, the government has to ensure that people know where to purchase masks and everyone can fairly purchase masks. At the same time, the government has to secure sufficient anti-epidemic materials for first-line anti-epidemic personnel in medical institutions. Therefore, the government immediately initiated the ban on the export of medical and activated carbon masks, requisitioned domestic mask-manufacturing capacity, and formed a national mask team to increase production capacity. Premier Su Tseng-Chang announced the implementation of the name-based medical mask distribution system on 3 February that makes it easier for people to purchase medical masks at the NHI-contracted pharmacies with their NHI card starting from 6 February and the NHIA was responsible for the establishment of the information system for contracted pharmacies.

That the NHI pharmacies were chosen as mask-selling locations is a testimony to the solid foundation that the NHI MediCloud System had built. In 2019, the network bandwidth among the medical institutions and the NHIA was originally upgraded from asymmetric digital subscriber line to a fiber network in response to medical image sharing. The upgraded network bandwidth is crucial for the name-based medical mask distribution system.

Pharmacists of the 6200 NHI-contracted pharmacies are already familiar with the NHI MediCloud System to check the medication information with patients' NHI cards to ensure the safety of the medication. The name-based medical mask distribution system was developed on the existing information operation mechanism. Although there were only 3 days for preparation, Dr. Lee, Director General of the NHIA, mobilized all divisions and tried his best to make people feel at ease about buying masks. The NHIA made a concise and simple introduction for the name-based medical mask distribution system and prepared the related Q&A; the regional divisions confirmed the computer operating environment of the pharmacy; data flow planning, program developing, information resource inventory, and adjustment were conducted by the division of information management. In addition, the connection between the regional divisions and the Federation of Taiwan Pharmacists Associations was used as a fast channel for two-way message transmission.

Government and Private Sectors Cooperate to Create the Mask Map

Originally, people could inquire about the address and phone number of the NHI-contracted pharmacies on the NHIA website. Before the name-based medical mask distribution system was launched, Audrey Tang, Minister without Portfolio, and her colleagues in the Executive Yuan were concerned about the planning situation of the NHIA's information system. The NHIA proposed that private communities may have access to the open datasets of the remaining number of masks. Audrey Tang's office strongly agreed with this idea and wanted to communicate with the private sectors.

On 5 February, the last day before launching the system, the NHIA provided the beta version of open datasets to the private community for system development and testing. Minister Tang and her colleague designed the Mask Supply and Demand Information Platform to compile links and instructions of the mask maps developed by the private sectors.

On the first day on which the name-based mask distribution policy was rolled out, more than 100 applications in the Mask Supply and Demand Information Platform were launched simultaneously. The open datasets were updated every 30 s by the NHIA, and these applications not only met the different usage habits and preferences of the user, but also dispersed the query system traffic. They also helped people to easily query various information such as the sales method, location, inventory of adults' or children's masks in various pharmacies, and choose a suitable place for purchasing. Improving the accessibility of masks was a great boost for policy promotion and was a model of advanced deployment.

Minister Tang mentioned in the online event "The Taiwan Model: When Civic Technology Meets Open Data" organized by the American Institute in Taiwan that this mask query application development transforms civic technology into civil engineering that everyone can use. It not only serves the public interest but allows participation from all sectors in Taiwan, which is exactly the connotation of the Taiwan Model.

The Coverage Rate of Name-Based Medical Mask Distribution System Is Improving Continuously

To solve the queuing and distribution problem in pharmacies and district public health centers and account for the difficulty of some office workers and students in buying masks during the business hours of pharmacies, in the weekly "Mask Policy Review Meeting" hosted by Premier Su, Minister Tang was appointed to coordinate the government, private industry, and information engineers who worked together to provide an online medical mask preorder system. The name-based medical mask distribution system 2.0 was launched on 12 March 2020. The public could log into the eMask website, the online medical mask preorder system, with an NHI card or a Citizen Digital Certificate. The NHI Express app also performed identity verification and connected to the eMask website.

My Health Bank system in the NHI Express app, which was designed to assist people in managing their own or family members' health, played an important role at that time. In May 2018, the NHIA launched the cell phone identification fast authentication to promote the My Health Bank system, and this application became the first choice of online identification function for the eMask system.

To make good use of the convenience store deeply embedded in Taiwanese culture, the name-based medical mask distribution system 3.0 was launched on 22

April to simplify the preorder process. People could insert their NHI cards to the kiosk as identification to preorder masks in more than 10,000 convenience stores and pay on-site. The mask system greatly reduced the cost of time queuing at the pharmacy.

The core value of the name-based mask rationing policy is fairness, which not only ensures the people's right to buy masks but also makes the material distribution more effective. As of 30 August 2020, approximately 21.6 million people had used the name-based medical mask distribution system, indicating that most people in Taiwan have used this service. It demonstrated the social value of fair distribution, as well as allowing all people to buy and wear masks correctly to assist in preventing the epidemic, which was one of the elements of Taiwan's successful epidemic prevention work at that time.

The Resilience of the NHIA Organization Is a Blessing For All

The NHI MediCloud System, the NHI Express app, the My Health Bank System, and other services combined with the NHI card have become an important mechanism for epidemic prevention. In July 2020, as the epidemic gradually eased, the government introduced a new epidemic prevention policy to activate the domestic economy, and the NHI card once again came in handy as a form of identification for purchasing Triple Stimulus Vouchers. In addition, in accordance with the concept of identity authentication for preordering masks, people can preorder Triple Stimulus Vouchers by using a kiosk in convenience stores, or the verification code generated by the NHI Express app, which disperses the crowds queuing at the post office effectively. The NHIA also provided the function such as querying the purchase records of masks and mask donation through NHI cards. The New Taiwan dollar (NTD) 500 sports vouchers and Art Fun Go Vouchers 2.0 launched by various ministries also apply the NHI card as a function of certification.

The NHI has been implemented in Taiwan for 27 years, and reformed and progressed along with the advancement of information technology. The single-payer insurance system was originally designed to take care of the health of the whole population. Under the trials of the pandemic, the NHIA adjusted the operation mechanism of the NHI and demonstrated its organizational resilience to shoulder the responsibility of epidemic prevention. Although the global pandemic continues to spread, Taiwan is one of the few places in the world that can maintain daily shopping and travel. The NHIA will continue to work seriously for the health of the all the people, and share the successful experience of Taiwan with the world, hoping that everyone globally will be able to overcome the difficulties of the pandemic together (Fig. 7.15).

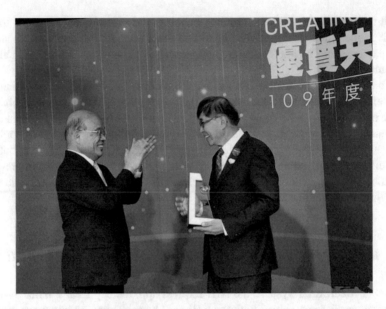

Fig. 7.15 In November 2020, the National Health Insurance Administration (NHIA) won the Open Data Award for its Mask Supply Information platform. Premier Su Tseng-Chang presented the award to NHIA Director General Lee

References

1. 20210718 自由共和國, Liberty Times Net.
2. 202012 Public Governance Quarterly.

Chapter 8
Drug and Medical Device Reimbursement

Hsueh-Yung (Mary) Tai

Introduction

Drug prices under the National Health Insurance (NHI) are important figures for the National Health Insurance Administration (NHIA) when reimbursing drug-related relevant expenses to medical institutions (Fig. 8.1).

As for medical devices, because the relative value unit (RVU) payments for items in the NHI Fee Schedule and Reference List for Medical Service already include the costs incurred by the medical devices and equipment in the medical process, they are not included in the Pharmaceutical Benefit and Reimbursement Scheme (PBRS).

The general public often only notices the adjustment of the drug price, the so-called "cutting the drug price." However, the determination and adjustment of the drug price and the coverage of medical devices in the NHI should be discussed in a holistic context. Therefore, we will explain and discuss the classification and price determination as well as the price adjustments of drug and medical devices.

How Are Drug Prices Determined?

The consideration factors for drugs to be listed under the NHI include relative medical benefits, cost-effectiveness, financial impact, and impact on medical ethics and social value. Drugs are categorized into new drugs, new items with the same active ingredients and dosage forms as those already listed under the NHI, and biosimilars (Fig. 8.2), and each category adopts different pricing methods.

H.-Y. (Mary) Tai (✉)
National Health Insurance Administration, Ministry of Health and Welfare, Taipei, Taiwan
e-mail: marytai@nhi.gov.tw

© The Author(s) 2022
P.-C. Lee et al. (eds.), *Digital Health Care in Taiwan*,
https://doi.org/10.1007/978-3-031-05160-9_8

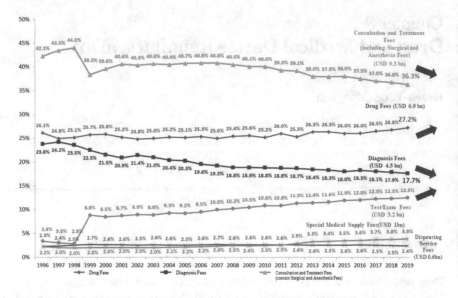

Fig. 8.1 Overview of medical expenditures

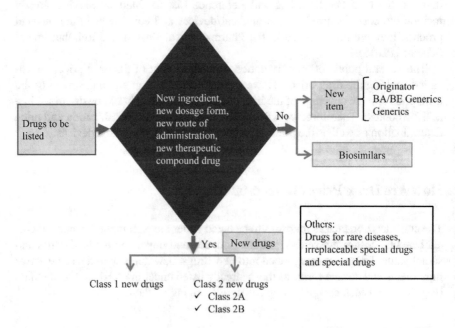

Fig. 8.2 Drug pricing process

Classification and Pricing of the Drugs Under the National Health Insurance

New drugs are classified as Class 1 new drugs with breakthrough innovations in medical value; Class 2A new drugs with moderate improvement in clinical value compared with the current best commonly used drugs; and Class 2B new drugs with clinical value similar to the drugs already included in the NHI. Class 1 new drugs are priced at the median drug price of 10 advanced (A-10) countries. Class 2 new drugs are capped at the median drug price of 10 A-10 countries, which are priced according to the lowest price in the A-10 countries, the drug price in the country of origin, the international drug price ratio of the new drug to the reference products, or the treatment-course dosage ratio of the new drug to the reference products.

For those conducting domestic clinical trials or pharmacoeconomic studies in Taiwan, up to 10% mark-up can be given in each case. When pricing by treatment-course dosage ratio method, mark-ups are given to those with better therapeutic effects, improved efficacy, enhanced safety, better convenience, or favorable dosage forms of children's medications (up to 15% for each criterium).

To encourage pharmaceutical companies conducting clinical trials and developing new drugs in Taiwan, a new drug that is first introduced in Taiwan and demonstrates significant clinical value, reduced adverse effects, or reduced drug resistance, is priced according to its actual transaction price, cost calculation method or the listing prices of A-10 countries of the new drugs and its comparators.

The new items are mostly generics. However, if a generic is listed first and its originator is listed later, then the originator becomes a "new item." The pricing principle of new items is mainly based on 80% or 90% (bioavailability/bioequivalence generic drug) of the price of the originator. For drugs that have been listed under the NHI for more than 15 years, as they are already off-patent, and considering that PIC/S GMP generics are requested to meet the same standard as the originators in terms of the quality of manufacturing, items with the same ingredient(s), dosage form, and specification are listed with the same price.

Biosimilars are priced at the lowest price among 85% of its listed originators, 85% of the A-10 median of its listed originator, 85% of the A-10 median of the biosimilar, and the price proposed by the drug supplier.

However, what is the reasonable price? Under the current NHI system, price adjustments are performed based on the transaction price at which drugs suppliers sell products to the medical institutions. The cost of a product and reasonable profit are also taken into consideration.

Adjustment of Drug Price

To review the prices of drugs that have come off patent for less than 5 years, drugs that have come off patent for less than 1 year are reviewed based on the A-10 reference price and market transaction situation. Those that have come off patent for more than 1 year but less than 5 years, are reviewed based on the market transaction situation. Other drugs are in principle adjusted based on the survey results of the market transaction. In addition, a lower limit on the adjusted drug prices is set to protect the listing price. The drug expenditure target (DET) has been implemented since 2013. Under the DET, drug prices are adjusted every year according to a preset target value, so that the adjustment range will be guaranteed (Fig. 8.3). For special drugs whose listing price is not high enough to cover the rising cost, pharmaceutical firms can propose to raise the listing price, so that their prices can be reviewed according to international prices or their costs and sent to the PBRS Joint Committee meeting for discussion.

The determination and adjustment of drug prices correlate closely with the dynamics in the drug market. Through 27 years of development and reform, the NHI has established a set of procedures for pricing and adjustment. In the future, as the insurer, the NHIA will continue to revise the methods and procedures for pricing and adjustment, with a view to providing reasonable drug prices and protecting the medication rights and benefits for patients.

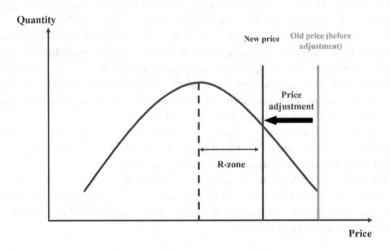

Fig. 8.3 Mechanism of drug price adjustment. Note: The NHIA obtains actual market transaction prices through regular drug price surveys and adjusts the listing prices of drugs based on the results of the survey

How to Classify Medical Devices and Determine the Price?

People often ask, what is the difference between medical devices and the NHI's special materials? How do we distinguish between them? And why can this one be included in the payment of the NHI, but that one can't? To put it simply, the definition of a medical device is specified in accordance with Article 13 of the Pharmaceutical Affairs Act, and is a product that has obtained a medical device license approved by the Taiwan Food and Drug Administration (TFDA) of the Ministry of Health and Welfare (MOHW). However, not all of them can be listed to be covered by the NHI. According to Article 3 of the NHI PBRS, the medical devices and special materials can be applied to the National Health Administration for a charge in addition to related treatment items and must be single-use medical devices that are not allowed to be reprocessed for a second use. Among them, the main items are "implants" or "temporary indwelling" medical devices and special materials. As of December 2020, the NHI has listed 1601 functional categories with 8228 items, which are mostly orthopedic materials, accounting for 35%, including bone screws, bone plates, artificial bones, artificial knee articular surface, and spinal fixators; second are cardiovascular medical devices, accounting for 24%, such as coronary artery balloon catheters, arterial vascular stents, artificial valves, and electrophysiology catheters; third are cannula medical devices and special materials accounting for 15%, such as infusion sets, catheters, and drainage catheters, whereas the rest are ophthalmology, embolization therapeutic materials, automatic suture nails, and vascular clips and needles.

Medical Devices and Special Material Classifications and Price Determinations

According to Article 3 of the PBRS, drug license holders or contracted institutions may apply to the National Health Administration to include MOHW-approved medical devices under NHI coverage. The application should be submitted with a TFDA-approved license and application form.

After collecting comprehensive information and a preliminary review, the application will first be reviewed by experts in a consultation meeting, and then submitted to the NHI PBRS Joint Committee. The medical devices will be listed as NHI-covered medical devices and special materials with the consensus of the representatives in the NHI PBRS Joint Committee.

The NHI's medical devices and special materials whose reimbursement prices are determined according to their function are divided into three types (Fig. 8.4).

1. New Items of Existing Function Categories

This type of medical device has the same function as the medical devices and special materials covered by the NHI, according to their effectiveness approved by

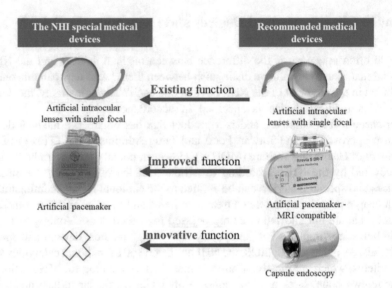

Fig. 8.4 The National Health Insurance medical devices and special materials are priced according to functional classification

the TFDA. The applicant should find similar NHI special medical devices as a reference by comparing function and effectiveness before submitting to the NHIA for reviewing. The initial reimbursement considering RVU verified by the NHI shall be determined to be the same as those of the same functional group in accordance with the National Health Insurance Act.

2. Medical Devices and Special Materials with New Function

These functional category items have not been listed in the NHI coverage before; they possess the "innovative function" or "improved function," which has more clinical value than existing NHI medical devices and special materials. After submitting clinical evidence and financial analysis review and evaluated by medical experts selected by the NHIA, the application will be submitted to an expert consultation meeting for discussion, and then to the NHI PBRS Joint Committee for further discussion and determination. The reimbursement price determination is in accordance with Articles 52, 52-1, 52-2, 52-3, and 52-4 of the PBRS, including the procurement price of public hospitals, medical centers (including would-be medical centers) or a combination of the two and dividing by the average of the RVU value with regard to the hospital global budget in the most recent four quarters, the self-paid price charged by medical institutions at all levels, the price in the United States, Australia, Japan, and South Korea, and considering the cost of the device.

Medical Devices and Special Materials Not Listed Independently or Not Covered

According to Article 3 of the PBRS, if the reimbursement payment has included surgery-relevant materials, treatment fees, anesthesia fees, examination fees, or the medical devices contained in the medical process, such as dressings, general sutures, blades, urinary catheters, nasogastric tubes, single-use medical devices used in procedures, testing reagents, and equipment, the NHI would no longer pay for them redundantly based on the principle of nonrepetitive payment.

According to Article 51 of the National Health Insurance Act, medical devices not required for positive therapies such as dentures, spectacles, and hearing aids are not covered by the NHI. In addition, Article 48 stipulates that the NHI does not pay for medical devices that are deemed to be non-essential for medical treatment or are evaluated as having a lack of economic benefits by the NHIA, or that do not meet the indications of the medical device license and the PBRS, or that do not have corresponding medical treatment. Therefore, if a new medical technology has no clinically corresponding treatment, the contracted institutions or medical associations should first apply to the NHIA for a new treatment item. In other words, the medical device can only be used after the relevant surgical methods or treatment are provided.

Amendment of Medical Devices and Special Materials and Adjustments to Reimbursement Payments

As medical technology advances, diagnosis and treatment technology improves, new types of medical equipment emerge, and clinical demands rise. If the payment regulations or the payment items do not meet the clinical needs, the medical device license holders, contracted medical institutions, or related medical associations can submit costs, clinical evidence, and other relevant information to the NHIA to propose amendments. The proposal is accepted after discussion and approval by the medical devices and special materials expert consultation meeting and the NHI PBRS Joint Committee.

If the clinically necessary or irreplaceable NHI medical devices or special materials cannot make ends meet owing to cost changes and other factors, and no supplier can provide the same functional items by the current NHI reimbursement payment, the medical device license holder can propose an adjustment to increase the NHI's reimbursement payment in accordance with Article 53-2 of the PBRS, and the additional add-on can be up to 10% considering reasonable factors. If the clinical needs cannot be met, contracted institutions and medical associations can also make the suggestion.

To establish an open, reasonable, and transparent payment adjustment system, and to shrink the difference between the reimbursement payment and the market price of medical devices, the NHIA conducts price and amount surveys in accordance with Articles 54 to 61 of the PBRS. This is to protect the rights and interests of those insured, stabilizing clinical supply and demand of medical devices and special materials, and making the payment more reasonable.

Perspective Control of Drug Costs Using the Drug Expenditure Target

The rationality of the drug prices and drug costs of the NHI has always been a concern to everyone. Since the introduction of the NHI, the drug costs have accounted for about 25% of overall medical expenses, which is generally higher than that of other countries. Before the second-generation NHI amendment, the NHIA conducted drug price surveys and adjustments every 2 years in accordance with the drug-price benchmarks to narrow the gap of between the payment of the NHI and the market transaction and bring the NHI drug price closer to market pricing.

Society has different opinions on biennial drug price adjustments, such as the drug price is not reduced enough, the adjustment interval is too long, the drug price is reduced too much, etc. After the second-generation NHI amendment, the MOHW listed the pilot program of the DET as a policy goal: to implement the overall drug cost control strategy, progress with transparency and predictability of the drug price adjustment system, and establish a resource allocation mechanism for NHI medical expenses. The NHIA announced the trial of the DET in 2013; by 2022 it had already been 10 years since its announcement.

Implementation of Overall Control of National Health Insurance Drug Prices

The pilot program implementation from 2013 to 2016 includes each global budget (excluding the Chinese medicine department), and the total growth rate of the global medical budget is adopted as the target growth rate. In response to external suggestions on the pilot program implementation of the DET, the NHIA has held many meetings to collect opinions from various sectors of society since 2017. After reviewing the pilot program, the scope of execution was revised to exclude the drugs expense from the medications of four types of diseases such as human immunodeficiency virus infection, hepatitis C, rare diseases, and hemophilia, and the growth rate of general service items was adopted. The refund of the price–volume agreement (PVA) is deducted when the target value of the drug expense is exceeded.

Implementation of the DET is used for determining the total drug price adjustments from a holistic viewpoint, and the drug price market surveys are used as the basis for adjusting individual drug prices. These are mainly for a preset "target

Table 8.1 Drug-price adjustments in drug expenditure targets (DET) over the years

Items	2013	2014	2015	2016	2017	2018	2019
Growth rate of the DET	4.528%	3.309%	3.481%	4.950%	4.280%	3.212%	4.080%
Target value (billion NTDs)	138.0	142.56	147.52	154.82	151.1	155.95	162.31
Payment (billion NTDs)	143.67	150.77	150.7	160.53	159.44	163.19	167.83
Excess quota (billion NTDs) & adjustment range	**5.67** (3.9%)	**8.21** (5.3%)	**3.18** (2.1%)	**5.71** (3.5%)	**7.382** (4.6%)	**5.83** (3.5%)	**4.04** (2.3%)
Starting date of new drug price	2014.5.1 2014.7.1	2015.4.1	2016.4.1	2017.4.1	2018.5.1	2019.4.1	2020.10.1

Note:
1. Since 2017, the medications for rare diseases, hemophilia, AIDS, and hepatitis C are not included in the DET, so the target value and payment exclude these expenses. From 2017, the "excess quota and adjustment range" is the payment minus the target value, and then the refund of the price volume agreement (PVA) is deducted.
2. In 2017, the refund of the PVA deducted was New Taiwan dollars (NTD) 0.958 billion; in 2018, the refund of PVA deducted was NTD 1.41 billion; in 2019, the refund of PVA deducted was NTD 1.48 billion.

value" of the annual drug expenditure, which is reviewed once a year, so that the drug expenditure can be maintained within a stable and reasonable range and linked with the actual drug expenses. When the target value is exceeded by the drug expenditure, the drug price adjustment will be automatically initiated in the next year. The NHIA keeps the system's overall spending on drugs stable and within a reasonable price by adjusting the drugs whose transaction prices have fallen, based on the survey results of drug market transactions and the amount exceeding the target value. Conversely, if the drug expenditure does not exceed the "target value," the drug price does not need to be adjusted. The drug-price adjustments in cooperation with the pilot program of the DET over the years are shown in Table 8.1.

Drug Expense Savings by the Joint Efforts of the Medical Profession, Pharmaceutical Profession, and the Public

The NHIA reviews whether the drug cost exceeds the target value annually and adjusts the unit drug price according to the amount exceeding the target value and the market transaction price. At the same time, we control the drug utilization more comprehensively, including professional review and reduction of refuse to reimburse indicators, monitoring of the number of drug items used in the outpatient, facilitation of integrated care plans, consulting for multiple medical consultations, and homecare visits by pharmacists to reduce the unnecessary drug utilization. National Health Insurance MediCloud System (NHI MediCloud System) was upgraded to reduce duplicated prescription of drugs of outpatients and to avoid drug-drug interactions. The NHIA provides the "Application Programming Interface" for the active reminder function of repetitive prescriptions across hospitals, which can provide real-time information on the remaining medicines of patients for doctors' reference in prescribing, and expanded the "Outpatient Drug Duplication Management Plan" from 12 categories to 60 from January 2019 and to all-oral medicines of the NHI from October 2019. To reduce the public concerns about drug wastage, the NHIA also actively aids the drug co-payment system to facilitate the cooperation of the medical profession, the pharmaceutical industry, and the public to save on pharmaceutical expenses.

Adjusting the prices of drugs that have been covered based on the results of competition in the drugs market, in addition to narrowing the drug-price gap, also slows down the growth of drug costs. In addition, it could further help to ensure reasonable RVUs for other medical services. In this way, patients in Taiwan can still use new drugs like advanced countries use under stable expenditures. It not only reduces people's out-of-pocket medical burden but also improves the quality of medical care, which will have substantial benefits for the whole healthcare system.

Drug Price Adjustments That Are More Transparent and Predictable

By setting the target value of drug expenditure in advance, and with the trend toward drug fee declaration and expenditure, the amount of the drug expenditure of the current year that may exceed the target value can be predicted ahead, which makes the adjustment of drug prices more transparent and predictable. However, if the excess amount of drug expenditure is used as the amount of drug-price adjustment, the difference between the excess amount and the actual transaction situation in the market is prone to occurring. For example, when the market price difference is large, only the amount exceeding the target expenditure can be adjusted owing to the restrictions of the system, which cannot effectively reflect the market transaction status and narrow the price difference. In addition, under the protection of the overall reduction of the DET, society has reported that some high-priced or high-cost drugs have a relatively small reduction and deviate greatly from international drug prices. It is necessary to carry out a further review with international drug prices as a supplement.

After the DET pilot program was launched, more than 7000 drug items were adjusted with the drug price each year. This is the most items with a one-time adjustment in the drug-price adjustment system, which has a great impact on the drug market of the NHI. After the price adjustment of drugs, there are also rumors that some drugs are withdrawn from the market of the NHI and that the price of a drug is cheaper than candy. However, adjusting the drug price of the NHI based on the market price of pharmaceutical manufacturers and account for the rights and interests of the people is a big challenge for the NHIA, so it sets a floor on the drug price. If the pharmaceutical manufacturers cannot make ends meet, they can submit the drug to be a special or irreplaceable special drug for a higher drug price, so as to deal with the concerns of the society about the drug-price adjustment. Through continuous communication and discussion of the DET, which is still currently a pilot program operation, it is hoped that the most suitable DET system for the NHI of Taiwan will be formed to ensure the long-term stability of the system and the maximum medical welfare of the people.

What Is the Managed Entry Agreement?

Owing to the aging of the population, the increment of chronic diseases and the continuous advancement of medical technology, expensive new drugs and new medical technologies have been launched one after another, and in particular, precision medicine has developed rapidly in recent years. These new medical technologies and new drugs cost a lot, which brings a heavy burden to the finances of the NHI. Since the inception of the NHI, medical expenses and drug expenditures have grown annually. The overall drug expenditures with a growth rate of 35.2% have grown from 154.1 billion RVUs in 2013 to 208.3 billion RVUs in 2019. The ratio of drug expenditures to medical expenses was 26.9% in 2019.

Drug Expenditures Grow Annually

In recent years, the financial balance of the NHI has faced significant challenges, and the payments deficit has gradually expanded under the limited growth in financial resources. To allocate the resources of the NHI fairly and to include new drugs in the reimbursement continuously so that all those insured can receive better health care, it is necessary to review the rationality of the overall drug payment structure. The price of old drugs is prevented from being higher than that of the new by appropriately reevaluating and reviewing the fee schedule of the old drugs that have been included in the NHI for many years.

The drug administration authorities of various countries have adopted an accelerated approval mechanism to speed up the launch of new drugs with unmet medical needs (such as new cancer drugs) in recent years. For patients' chance of survival, various countries have replaced objective indicators of overall survival with surrogate indicators such as progression-free survival, tumor shrinkage, or others, hoping to shorten the time for observation and research and accelerate the launch of drugs. However, it increases the uncertainties in clinical effects, cost-effectiveness, and the financial impact, so that the NHIA needs to further monitor after the listing of a new drug. Countries such as the United Kingdom, Italy, Canada, and South Korea have adopted risk-sharing mechanisms to solve these problems.

Formulating Multiple Risk-Sharing Mechanisms

Taiwan is also facing the same problem at present. With the rapid research and development technologies of drugs, many patients are looking forward to various new drugs launched one after another. However, new drugs are expensive, but the actual clinical efficacy is highly uncertain. For instance, it is still not clear which cancer drugs are effective in which patient groups. When considering whether to include the new drug in the NHI's reimbursements, it is necessary to carefully evaluate the cost-effectiveness and whether they are worthy or not. To improve the accessibility of new drugs to patients, and to solve the problems regarding uncertainties in efficacy and financial impact, the MOHW, referring to foreign practices, announced the amendment of the "Pharmaceutical Benefit and Reimbursement Schedule" on 19 September 2018 to add Managed Entry Agreement (MEA)-related regulations, and formulate multiple risk-sharing mechanisms for reimbursement (Table 8.2). MEAs include multiple methods such as pharmaceutical firms returning a certain percentage of the drug fee based on the patient's overall survival, progression-free survival, and clinical efficacy after setting the drug price, or the pharmaceutical firms provide a fixed discount to subsidize treatment and part of the drug fee of the co-prescribed drugs, so that the NHIA and pharmaceutical firms can use these methods together when negotiating drug payment. The NHIA and pharmaceutical firms share the risk of financial uncertainty arising from high-cost drugs. If the clinical efficacy of the new drug is not significantly better than that of the traditional drug, the pharmaceutical firms must repay, reduce the price, or share the cost together according to the contract, which will assist in accelerating the introduction of the new drug.

In addition, the provisions also clearly state that pharmaceutical firms have to provide empirical evaluation data on the efficacy of drugs with the MEA within a certain period for the NHIA to review the relevant regulations on drug payment and the price to increase the appropriateness and account for the rights and safety of drug utilization for patients.

Table 8.2 Managed Entry Agreement (MEA) models

Categories of the MEA	Model content
1. Agreement based on *performance*	1. Ensure the improvement in overall survival 2. Ensure progression-free survival 3. Refund/payback based on clinical performance
2. Agreement based on the *financial results*	1. Refund/payback 2. Free doses 3. Payback for co-prescribed drugs
3. Agreement based on the *sharing mechanisms*	Mutual share of refund/payback among pharmaceutical products with the same ingredient or pharmacological category

Using Health Technology Reassessment to Improve the Benefits of Drug and Medical Device Payments

How to improve the reasonable use of medical resources is an important issue for the NHI of Taiwan at this stage. With limited medical resources, the aging population, and the introduction of high-tech medical care, the medical expenses of the NHI in Taiwan are increasing rapidly. In addition, with the advancement of research and development in health technology, some of the listed products are no longer cost effective.

To improve the reasonable use of medical resources, all countries in the world are currently advocating the establishment of regulations and mechanisms for the Health Technology Reassessment (HTR). Countries including Australia, Spain, South Korea, and the Netherlands have established related mechanisms for the HTR. Implementation of the HTR is mainly to systematically transfer resources from low-efficiency health technology to high-efficiency interventional measures and health technology through continuous monitoring and tracking the listed products. It allows reallocation of medical resources to achieve maximum efficiency and ensures that health technology can be utilized in the most appropriate ways. By reassessing the health technologies, products may maintain their reimbursement status and be subject to restriction or expansion of reimbursement regulations, or delisting.

To reduce the financial burden and be in line with international practices, and considering that Article 72 of the NHI Act stipulates that "To reduce cases of ineffective treatment and other inappropriate use of insurance medical resources, the Insurer shall draft an annual proposal for controlling inappropriate use of resources; present it to the National Health Insurance Committee (NHIC) for discussion, and submit it to the Competent Authority afterwards for approval," the NHIA has been working on establishing a domestic "HTR mechanism" since 2018. By collecting and analyzing the experience of Australia, South Korea, the Netherlands, and Spain with the HTR, we aim to establish a systematic review mechanism for tracking and monitoring the efficacy and cost-effectiveness of the listed products. The mechanism initially developed is as follows (Fig. 8.5).

The items already listed account for most of the NHI resources, whereas new health technology only accounts for a small part of it. Therefore, facing the burden of limited medical resources, the efficiency regarding the reimbursement of the listed products needs to be urgently reevaluated. In the future, the NHIA will continue to discuss with relevant sectors to establish a domestic "HTR mechanism" and modify the reimbursed indications and criteria according to the evaluation results, to achieve the optimal use and rational allocation of medical resources.

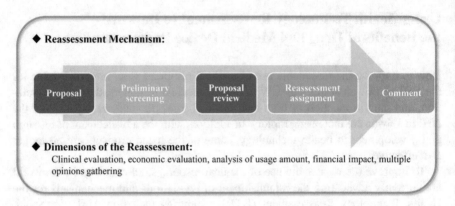

Fig. 8.5 Health Technology Reassessment mechanism. Notes: The dimensions of the reassessment will be adjusted based on the items.

Using Real-World Data to Evaluate the Payment Effects of Drugs and Medical Devices in Taiwan

In recent years, real-world data (RWD)-driven real-world evidence has been widely used to evaluate the safety and efficacy of post-marketing medical products. The NHIA has also established an RWD-collecting platform during the process of the NHI covering drugs and medical devices. This platform uses real-world evidence to analyze and evaluate the benefits of reimbursed products by collecting information regarding the real use and claims, uploaded examination results and reports, medical image data, and other NHI big data. This will compensate for the limitations of traditional randomized clinical trials in drug research and development and the dilemma of insufficient clinical evidence for medical devices. In this way, medical resources are appropriately used for patient sharing in different departments to achieve the goal of improving the quality of medical care and protecting the people's health and well-being.

Monitoring Efficacy of Hemophilia Treatment

Hemophilia is an inherited bleeding disorder caused by deficiency in coagulation factors. Hemophilia A and B are the most common types of hemophilia, with deficiency in factor VIII and factor IX respectively. The disease status of hemophilia can be classified into mild, moderate, or severe depending on the concentration of the patients' coagulation factor.

Preventing and treating the bleeding caused by insufficient coagulation factors is the major treatment target for hemophilia. Supplementary coagulation factors are given to the patients to maintain the normal function of muscles and joints. However, a certain percentage of the patients under the treatment will develop antibodies against the coagulation factors, resulting in a decline in efficacy. It is necessary to adjust current treatments or choose appropriate alternative treatments for patients with anti-coagulation factor antibodies based on the antibody titer, clinical response to the drugs, and the cause and site of bleeding. Therefore, in the treatment of hemophilia, it is essential to monitor the efficacy as well as patients' response to medication in a timely fashion and take a blood test regularly to monitor coagulation factor concentration and antibody level, to ensure that the treatment achieves the best outcome.

The medications for hemophilia are very expensive, but the life expectancy and quality of life of patients with hemophilia are similar to those of the general population because of the advancement of medical care. The care for hemophilia has also been advancing toward patient-centered care instead of merely giving medications to prevent bleeding and on-demand treatment upon bleeding or surgery. In addition, owing to the continuous introduction of new coagulation factor agents and high-priced new drugs, the expenditure and the financial impact of hemophilia treatment are increasing.

To improve the treatment outcome of hemophilia, reduce the wastage of resources, and optimize the benefits of limited medical resources, the NHIA has amended the reimbursement regulations and developed a "hemophilia case management system" to strengthen the monitoring and evaluation of the actual medication use and treatment outcomes of patients with hemophilia. This system includes complete information regarding treatment, diagnosis, medication monitoring, antibody examination, and efficacy to understand the real-world efficacy and strengthen the rational use of drugs. The relevant information is not only for physicians to make follow-up treatment evaluations based on medication and treatment outcomes, but also for the revision of overall hemophilia patient care policies and payment regulations.

Evaluation of Medication Use for Rare Diseases

Because of the high price of drugs and the small patient population in terms of rare diseases, the National Health Administration has been planning to use RWD for evaluation after listing.

Spinraza has been reimbursed in Taiwan since 1 July 2020. Its reimbursement regulation stipulates that patients shall register on the registry system, monitor regularly, and upload the evaluation result. It is also necessary to close the case in the system once the treatment is over or when a patient stops using the drug.

Rolling Evaluation of Cancer Immunotherapy

To satisfy patients' expectations of receiving new drug treatments early, the NHIA is constantly trying to strike a balance between payment and financial impact. In 2019, the NHIA adopted an approach of paying first and the reassessing, and to list cancer immunotherapy used for eight cancers and 11 indications approved by the MOHW. Taiwan's NHI has listed certain cancer immunotherapies earlier than other countries. The NHIA then implemented the rolling evaluation to review the reimbursed indications based on the scientific evidence for the patients' actual response to medication.

After a year of RWD collection, the NHIA found that the overall response to drugs for cancer immunotherapy, the complete/partial response (CR/PR), was 20–30% on average. It shows that the relative benefit was limited. The survival rates of patients treated with immunotherapy, chemotherapy, or targeted therapy are similar in patients with gastric cancer and liver cancer. The therapeutic effect may not be better, but the NHI has to afford the cost of drugs several times. Therefore, the PBRS Joint Committee decided to suspend applications from new cases, but the medication can be extended by up to 2 years for patients with a better response.

Evaluation of New Oral Drugs for Hepatitis C

To know the actual efficacy of new oral drugs for hepatitis C after these drugs were covered by the NHI, the NHIA has requested medical institutions to register the patients' viral amount after treatment. Analyzing the cases with viral amount 12 weeks after the end of medication from 2017 to 2019, 96.9%, 97.4%, and 98.7% of the cases had undetectable viral amounts respectively. The average treatment success rate is 98.1%, which is quite high.

Evaluation of Long-Term Ventricular Assist System

Furthermore, the NHIA also uses RWD for medical devices with higher financial impact or uncertain efficacy. For example, the payment for "long-term ventricular assist device (VAD)" covered by NHI since October 2018 was 4.25 million RVUs. As of October 2018 to May 2020, 31 patients in the database all survived, and 5 of them underwent heart transplantation within 1 year after installing a VAD, with a cumulative incidence of about 22%. There were records of two complication, which mainly happened in the first 3 months after installing the device, with a cumulative incidence of no complications of 92%. A total of 21 patients were annotated with New York Heart Association (NYHA) heart function classification indicators. After the long-term VAD was installed, the NYHA function level of all patients improved. In addition, the proportion of patients with NYHA I and NYHA II after installing the device was 95.2% of the overall patients.

Evaluation of Transcatheter Aortic Valve Implantation

At present, the payment for transcatheter aortic valve implantation covered by the NHI since 1 February 2021, is 1.09 million RVUs. An RWD platform has also been established to facilitate the collection of RWD in Taiwan and to analyze the clinical benefit after the medical device covered by the NHI as a basis for the reevaluation of the benefits of payments.

The belief of the NHI is reasonable payment for "valuable" drugs, medical devices, and medical services and striving for the rights and interests of patients under affordable finance. The NHIA will uphold the belief in caring for patients and promote precision medicine based on evidence-based medicine. We look forward to working with patients to achieve the best benefits of payments for medical devices.

Horizon Scanning for Budgeting New Drugs

In recent years, the drug market has made breakthroughs in the development of many new cancer drugs owing to the investment of many drug companies in research and development. There are more and more treatment options for cancer patients, but the cost of new drugs is expensive, and the burden on the drug expenditures of governments of various countries will become much heavier. To safeguard the rights and interests of patients' medication, meet the clinical needs of patients, fully comply with international treatment standards, and ensure the sustainability of high-quality medical care, the NHIA has endeavored to introduce various new drugs in recent years. The proportion of cancer drugs increased year by year from 2018 to 2020. To ensure the sustainability of the NHI and patients' rights in the use of medication, how to allocate a high enough budget for new drugs has become an important issue.

To make the estimated new drug budget closer to the actual amount required, the NHIA referred to the UK and Canada's approach to establishing the Horizon Scanning mechanism, and held a meeting with the industry, government, and academia on 9 September 2020. On 13 October of the same year, experts around the world were invited to share their experience. It is hoped that the Horizon Scanning mechanism could be a reference for the annual new drug budget preparation.

The NHIA completed and officially launched the "Budget Estimated Registration and Platform for Horizon Scanning New Drugs and New Benefit Scope" system on 30 September 2020. Pharmaceutical firms can register information about new drugs expected to enter the market on the platform. Taking the compilation of a new drug budget for 2022 as an example, pharmaceutical firms filled in the new drug-related information expected to be listed in 2021 and 2022 on the platform before 30 November 2020, including drug name (in Chinese and English), ingredient name, dosage form, strength, budget category (general or special), the declared value of the new drug, expected year and month of market launch, expected indication, expected proposal submission date, expected reimbursed indications, expected date of listing, proposed listing price, pricing comparators, estimated patient population, financial forecast, estimated replacement, budget impact, etc.

To resolve the uncertainties in the budget, the NHIA continues to revise the estimation mechanism of the new drug budget and refer to the opinions of all parties. In recent years, the average value of the declared drug fees for new drugs listed in the past 5 years was used as the budgetary increase in new drugs after excluding the substitution effect. The Horizon Scanning evaluation operations have been developed considering that the rapid development of new drug technology, the types of new drugs included each year, and the payment prices of products are very different. It is hoped that by collecting and estimating the budget required for the expected drugs in advance, budgeting for drugs in the future will be more precise, the financial impact of the NHI can be reduced, and the rights and interests of patients in drug use can be protected.

Conclusion

The rationality of the medical costs of the NHI has always been a topic of concern to everyone. After much time in development and reform, the determination and adjustment of the NHI's prices for drugs and medical devices have been developed with an associated set of procedural steps for pricing. Through the DET, MEA, and other measures, the NHIA strives not only to allocate the resources fairly but also to include new drugs in the reimbursement continuously. Through relevant laws and regulations, there are also procedures for medical devices with new technologies, which are needed clinically, to be covered by the NHI. To provide better health care for all those insured, the NHIA will continuously refine the system for the payment and inclusion of drugs and the medical devices.

Chapter 9
Coverage of Advanced Treatments and Medical Devices

Hsueh-Yung (Mary) Tai and Yu-Pin Chang

Introduction

With the development of the medical industry, immunotherapy brings a new dawn for cancer treatment, and personalized precision medicine has been applied in the development of cancer treatment with the advancement of molecular medicine (Fig. 9.1).

Owing to advancements in treatment, Taiwan, with a high prevalence of hepatic cirrhosis, aims to expand the reimbursement indications in hepatitis B and strives to eradicate hepatitis C by 2025.

In addition, as the treatment pattern has changed from traditional surgeries in the past to interventional treatment, endoscopic surgery, and robotic arms, plus the increasing life expectancy of the national people, the clinical and public demand for new medical devices has been growing.

In this chapter, we will discuss the rationale and the decision-making process of combining reimbursement of advanced treatments (immuno-oncology therapy, hepatitis B and C medications), tests (next-generation sequencing, NGS), and medical devices in the benefits package of the National Health Insurance (NHI).

H.-Y. (Mary) Tai (✉) · Y.-P. Chang
National Health Insurance Administration, Ministry of Health and Welfare, Taipei, Taiwan
e-mail: marytai@nhi.gov.tw; A110413@nhi.gov.tw

© The Author(s) 2022
P.-C. Lee et al. (eds.), *Digital Health Care in Taiwan*,
https://doi.org/10.1007/978-3-031-05160-9_9

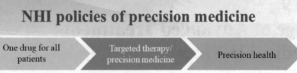

Including Immuno-oncology Therapy in National Health Insurance Benefits

To enable cancer patients to be treated with new drugs as soon as possible, cancer immunotherapy for eight cancer types and 11 indications have been covered by the NHI since 2019, such as the first-line treatments for nonsmall-cell lung cancer and urothelial carcinoma, earlier than other Asian countries. Then, the reimbursed indications were reviewed according to the scientific evidence of the patients' real-world treatment outcome. Based on the evaluation results, since 2020, the reimbursed course of treatment was determined to extend up to 2 years for patients responsive to the medication. As for the gastric and liver cancer indications, as it shows no significant benefits compared with the existing treatments, for the first time the National Health Insurance Administration (NHIA) decided to suspend applications from new patients because the drug supplier didn't agree on the risk-sharing scheme, but patients who are already under the treatment can continue until disease progression.

Immunotherapy is a trend in cancer treatment. Since April 2019, the NHI has covered cancer immunotherapy, including pembrolizumab, nivolumab, atezolizumab, and avelumab for the treatment of melanoma, nonsmall-cell lung cancer, classic Hodgkin's lymphoma, urothelial carcinoma, head and neck squamous cell carcinoma, gastric adenocarcinoma, renal cell carcinoma, hepatocellular carcinoma, Merkel Cell Carcinoma, and other indications. Patients who meet the criteria of PD-L1 expression are fully covered by the NHI.

Because some indications of the cancer immunotherapy have not yet completed phase III clinical trials, the clinical benefits are uncertain. To let the patients who can really benefit use the drug, the registry system for "Pre-Review of Cancer Immunotherapy Case Applications" has been established since the cancer immunotherapy was first listed. This system collects real-world data (RWD) such as the treatment outcomes and significant adverse effects of patients under the treatment, so that the benefits and rationality of the payment for such drugs could be evaluated.

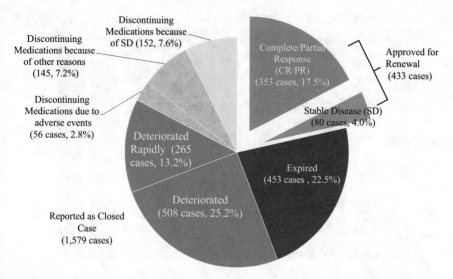

Fig. 9.2 Analysis of the outcomes of the latest treatment in patients using cancer immunotherapy. Note: (1) Cases for analysis: 2012 cases that have been approved for renewal. (2) As of 30 September 2020

According to the results of real-world evidence (RWE) analysis, the response rate to cancer immunotherapy, including complete/partial response (CR/PR), is only about 20% on average (Fig. 9.2). Although the relative benefits are limited, to let patients responsive to the treatment benefit from the value of the new drugs, the NHIA decided that since April 2020, patients who have been evaluated as having stable disease after treatment can continue the treatment for another 12 weeks, the same as those with CR/PR. In the mean time, the reimbursed course of treatment is extended up to 2 years for patients responsive to the treatment; as for patients with urothelial carcinoma with a relatively good response rate, the reimbursement criteria are also loosened.

On the other hand, more than 90% of gastric cancer patients and about 80% of liver cancer patients did not respond to cancer immunotherapy drugs (Fig. 9.3). Although the treatment outcomes differ between patients treated by different physicians, most patients experienced disease progression or expired within about 2 months after the treatment. The treatment outcomes are similar to those of patients treated with chemotherapy or target therapy, but the NHI has to pay several times more. Therefore, after referring to domestic data, international cancer treatment guidelines, and other reimbursement recommendations from the United Kingdom, Australia, and Canada, the National Health Insurance Pharmaceutical Benefit and Reimbursement Scheme Joint Committee, which is composed of professionals, representatives of medical associations, employers, and patient groups, decided to suspend applications from new patients with these two cancers, but patients who are already under treatment can continue the treatment until disease progression.

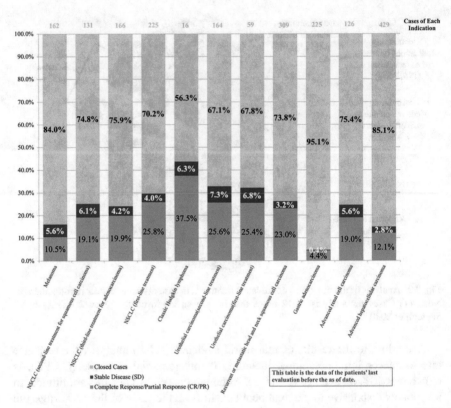

Fig. 9.3 The latest evaluation of disease status in each indication. Note: (1) Cases for analysis: 2012 cases that have been approved for renewal. (2) As of 30 September 2020

To provide patients with gastric cancer and liver cancer with new treatment options, the NHIA continues to communicate with pharmaceutical firms on diversified reimbursement mechanisms, hoping that pharmaceutical firms can share the drug costs for patients not responsive to the treatment, and ask pharmaceutical firms to develop precise pretreatment testing methods to find out patients suitable for treatments and ensure the safe use of medications. At the same time, the NHIA also speeds up the relaxation of the reimbursement regulations for other treatments used for gastric and liver cancer, such as expanded coverage of Herceptin and Lonsurf for gastric cancer treatment and the listing of the targeted therapy for liver cancer, Lenvima, hoping to provide patients with more beneficial treatment options.

Since the listing of cancer immunotherapy in 2019, more than 3200 patients have applied to use the medication, reflecting the medical needs of patients. The NHIA also continues to collect patients' responses to the medication as suggested by cancer patient groups, hoping to use RWD to evaluate and review the reimbursement regulations of cancer immunotherapy. To ensure cancer immunotherapy use in patients who can benefit from the medication, the NHI has also covered four types of PD-L1 kits for pretreatment testing since April 2020. This helps to identify patients who are likely responsive to cancer immunotherapy and enhances reimbursement efficiency.

Owing to the accelerated market approval process of new cancer drugs in many countries, the clinical benefits of cancer immunotherapy become highly uncertain, resulting in most public insurance schemes facing the risk of financial impact. Despite limited resources, Taiwan's NHI covers cancer immunotherapy by adopting risk-sharing mechanisms and uses the RWE collected from the registry for evaluation, which can serve as references for decision-making and revising reimbursement regulations. This helps to enhance the efficiency of reimbursement. This reimbursement model can be applied to the listing of more new cancer drugs in the future. It enhances patient access to new drugs and allows pharmaceutical firms to share the risk of financial impact, which helps to ensure the sustainability of the NHI.

Inclusion of Next-Generation Sequencing in National Health Insurance Benefits

In the past, cancer drug treatment followed empirical therapy based on the accumulated clinical data from patients. Patients with the same type of cancer and cancer staging were given the same treatment, and doctors tried to control tumors with various drugs. They first gave drug A for treatment and then changed to drug B if the efficacy of drug A was low. With the advancement of molecular medicine, personalized precision medicine has been applied in the development of cancer treatment, enabling each patient's specific biomarkers to be considered when determining the corresponding treatment. For example, only lung adenocarcinoma patients with epidermal growth factor receptor (EGFR) mutations would be given EGFR-targeted drugs to provide patients with a more effective and personalized treatment. Besides relieving the patients from suffering illness caused by traditional trial treatments, personalized medicine would reduce unnecessary examinations, tests, and consultation for the NHI.

Individual Genetic Testing

Currently, the genetic testing items covered by the NHI are single-gene tests carried out one after another according to the incidence of genetic mutations. Taking lung cancer as an example, EGFR and anaplastic lymphoma kinase (ALK) mutations, two common mutations in lung cancer patients, which account for 50% of the mutations, are tested first, and then the remaining specimen will be tested for other possible genes. However, the sequential test method may cause the risk of an

Table 9.1 Molecular diagnosis for cancer precision (excluding out-of-pocket costs and manufacturer's repayments)

Testing item	Payment starting date	Paid RVUs	2019			2020		
			Cases	Times of test	RVU of test (million RVUs)	Cases	Times of test	RVU of test (million RVUs)
Cytogenetics	1 March 1995	11,871	7933	10,124	119.74	8280	10,979	129.79
Her-2/neu ISH	1 January 2009	10,400	3778	4279	43.34	4088	4705	47.91
RQ-PCR for leukemia	1 December 2015	3571	2771	8403	28.29	3211	10,464	35.31
EGFR mutation (IVD)	1 June 2019	8252	4585	4781	38.64	8800	9199	74.81
EGFR mutation (LDT)	1 September 2019	6755	171	172	1.16	467	478	3.23
DNA qualitative amplification test	1 July 2014	1000	76,095	160,332	157.77	85,846	227,875	224.05
RNA qualitative amplification test	1 July 2014	1200	31,567	74,245	92.45	78,228	192,562	242.33
DNA quantitative amplification test	1 July 2014	2000	160,684	297,428	558.43	170,203	327,501	617.27

ISH in situ hybridization, *RQ-PCR* real-time quantitative polymerase chain reaction, *EGFR* epidermal growth factor receptor, *IVD* in vitro diagnostics, *RDT* rapid diagnostic test

unsatisfactory specimen, resulting in repeated specimen collection and delays in the timing of treatment.

According to statistics of the nine genetic testing items covered by the NHI (Table 9.1), leukemia, breast cancer, and lung cancer testing contribute to the majority of the testing costs, reaching 1.48 billion to 1.69 billion relative value units (RVUs) from 2019 to 2020 (excluding out-of-pocket costs and manufacturer's repayments). The ALK in vitro diagnostics testing, an immunohistochemistry method for lung cancer, and All-RAS (rat sarcoma) mutation testing for colorectal cancer have been approved by the "National Health Insurance Fee Schedule and Reference List for Medical Services Joint Committee" in 2020. After agreements with pharmaceutical companies are signed, revising the fee schedule for these genetic tests and corresponding targeted therapy will be concurrently effective.

Future Direction: Next-Generation Sequencing

Next-generation sequencing, also known as second-generation sequencing, refers to methods different from the low throughput, high-cost, and time-consuming Sanger sequencing. Because NGS could process a larger number of nucleic acids simultaneously, its advantages, such as low cost of single-base sequencing, high throughput, and high speed, break the limitation of gene size or number for gene sequencing.

In response to the trend toward personalized precision medicine, the NHIA has begun to compile the list of targeted therapies that have been reimbursed by NHI or that will become covered shortly and their corresponding genetic testing. Questions and challenges regarding covering NGS as a treatment item are under discussion as well. For example, what is included in the list of genes that need to be sequenced for clinical practice? The cost calculation and test report format for NGS are also waiting to be determined.

Biotechnology industry laboratories are currently performing most NGS. However, according to Article 27, Paragraph 1 of the "Regulations Governing Contracting and Management of National Health Insurance Medical Care Institutions" and Note 33 of the "Report Format and Filling Instructions of Outpatient Medical Expenses of Contracted Medical Service Institutions," hospitals can only entrust NHI-contracted medical institutions with performing medical examinations. Therefore, the NHI must review the feasibility of contracted hospitals entrusting external laboratories with the Laboratory Developed Test without violating current medical regulations and start drafting the expansion of the coverage and revising the fee schedule for the Laboratory Developed Test.

Expansion of the Coverage of Medications to Eradicate Hepatitis B and C

The World Health Organization (WHO) has proposed the goal of eliminating viral hepatitis by 2030, including a 90% reduction of new cases of chronic viral hepatitis B and C infections, 65% reduction of viral hepatitis B and C deaths, and treating 80% of eligible patients with chronic hepatitis B and C virus infection, aiming to stop the transmission of viral hepatitis. Therefore, the NHI plays an important role in providing patients with affordable and effective treatment.

Why Is the Treatment of Viral Hepatitis So Important?

Hepatitis B and C are important factors leading to liver cirrhosis and liver cancer. 15–20% of hepatitis B carriers with chronic hepatitis will develop liver cirrhosis, and cirrhosis will increase the incidence of liver cancer. More than half of hepatitis

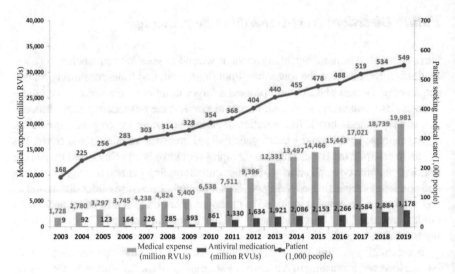

Fig. 9.4 Statistics on hepatitis B patients over the years. Note: The data include outpatient and inpatient cases with hepatitis B-related diagnoses in the claimed primary and secondary diagnosis codes

C infected patients will develop chronic hepatitis, and about 20% of them will develop liver cirrhosis, and every year about 3–5% of patients with liver cirrhosis will get liver cancer.

According to the analysis of the top 10 causes of death in Taiwan in 2019, chronic liver disease and liver cirrhosis are the tenth cause of death, and liver cancer is the second cause of cancer death. According to the claims data of the NHI, the number of hepatitis B patients has increased from nearly 168,000 in 2003 to 549,000 in 2019, and the RVUs of hepatitis B have also increased from 1.72 billion to 19.98 billion, which is an increase of nearly 12-fold in 17 years (Fig. 9.4). The expenditure on hepatitis B oral antiviral agents was 3.18 billion RVUs, which accounts for only 16%, and the remaining direct or indirect medical expenses account for 84%. As for hepatitis C, the number of patients has increased from nearly 74,000 in 2003 to 205,000 in 2019, and the RVUs of hepatitis C have also increased from 1.38 billion to 17.39 billion, which is an increase of nearly 13-fold in 17 years (Fig. 9.5). In the year before the new direct-acting antiviral agents for hepatitis C were covered, expenditure on antiviral medications used for the treatment of hepatitis C only accounted for 8.4%, and expenditure on other direct or indirect treatment accounted for 91.6%.

From the above data, we can understand that if hepatitis is not well controlled, liver cirrhosis and liver cancer will increase. If hepatitis patients can receive antiviral medication and be controlled properly, the NHI resources used to treat liver cirrhosis and liver cancer can also be saved for the treatment of other diseases. Based on this principle, the reimbursement indications for hepatitis B and hepatitis C

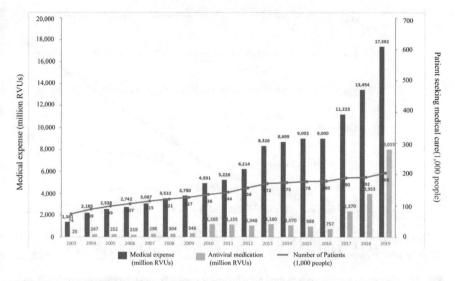

Fig. 9.5 Statistics on hepatitis C patients over the years. Note: The data include outpatient and inpatient cases with hepatitis C-related diagnoses in the claimed primary and secondary diagnosis codes

medications in the NHI have also been gradually expanding along with the latest clinical developments.

Treatment of Hepatitis B Medication Under National Health Insurance

Taiwan began to promote the viral hepatitis treatment plan in 2003, and about 3000 people were treated with hepatitis B medication in the same year. Along with the progress in research, the NHI has gradually expanded the coverage according to the treatment guidelines for hepatitis B. From 2003 to 2019, the number of patients who have received hepatitis B medication was approximately 211,000 (Fig. 9.6). If 545,000 hepatitis B patients require treatment, the coverage rate of hepatitis B patients receiving treatment is 38.7% (211,000 ÷ 545,000).

As for the reimbursed medications for hepatitis B medication, it has been gradually expanding over the years. The key points are summarized below.

1. November 2009: the treatment course covered by the NHI was extended from at most 18 months to 36 months (for those with hepatitis B e-antigen (HBeAg) test turning negative during the treatment course, they can be paid for another 12 months).

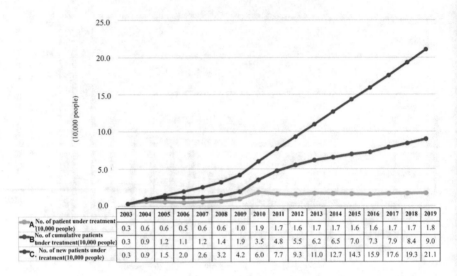

	2003	2004	2005	2006	2007	2008	2009	2010	2011	2012	2013	2014	2015	2016	2017	2018	2019
A No. of patient under treatment (10,000 people)	0.3	0.6	0.6	0.5	0.6	0.6	1.0	1.9	1.7	1.6	1.7	1.7	1.6	1.6	1.7	1.7	1.8
B No. of cumulative patients under treatment(10,000 people)	0.3	0.9	1.2	1.1	1.2	1.4	1.9	3.5	4.8	5.5	6.2	6.5	7.0	7.3	7.9	8.4	9.0
C No. of new patients under treatment(10,000 people)	0.3	0.9	1.5	2.0	2.6	3.2	4.2	6.0	7.7	9.3	11.0	12.7	14.3	15.9	17.6	19.3	21.1

Fig. 9.6 The number of patients treated with National Health Insurance-covered hepatitis B antiviral medications

2. July 2010:

    (a) Long-term coverage of liver cirrhosis.
    (b) The reimbursed treatment course extends from 2 years to 3 years for those who develop resistance to the first-line treatment. If they relapse after medication withdrawal, patients can be treated with the combination therapy once, and the course of treatment is 3 years.

3. January 2017

    (a) HBeAg positive before treatment: treatment until HBeAg turns negative and then another 12 months of coverage.
    (b) HBeAg negative before treatment: at least 2 years of the treatment course, and HBV DNA is tested every 6 months during the treatment for a total of three times. Withdraw the medication if the HBeAg tests are all negative, and the maximum reimbursement period is 36 months each time.
    (c) To cancel the limit (used to be twice per patient) on the number of treatments.

4. February 2018: highly infectious pregnant women with hepatitis B are covered from the 28th week of pregnancy to 4 weeks after delivery, further reducing the risk of vertical infection.

5. March 2021: the NHIA invited gastroenterologists to discuss the revision of the reimbursement regulations for hepatitis B medication, and there are five major points as follows:

    (a) Revise the reimbursement criteria for initiating therapy in patients with the signs of virus replication and active hepatitis.
    (b) Revise the reimbursement criteria for long-term treatment of liver cirrhosis.

(c) Revise the reimbursement criteria for pre-exposure prophylaxis in nonliver transplant recipients.
(d) Revise the reimbursement criteria for initiating therapy in patients of liver cancer who can receive eradicative treatment.
(e) Newly added reimbursement criteria for treatment and prevention of hepatitis B in patients receiving immunosuppressant treatment.

Treatment of Hepatitis C Under the National Health Insurance

In the past, treatment for hepatitis C involved using pegylated interferon once a week combined with daily oral ribavirin, and the treatment took 6 months to 1 year. However, because interferon has to be injected frequently and the side effects are obvious, patients are discouraged from receiving the treatment, which results in a low treatment rate for hepatitis C. By the end of 2017, there were about 95,000 hepatitis C patients receiving interferon treatment, which is still lower than the number of people infected in Taiwan. Since 2014, direct-acting antiviral agents with a high cure rate have been successively launched around the world. The new direct-acting antiviral agents only need to be taken for 2–4 months, reducing side effects, and the cure rate is more than 90%.

In response to the trend toward hepatitis C patients receiving new drug treatments, the budget allocation and priority of the treatment population have become an important issue. The NHIA held the "Public Hearings of Hepatitis C Treatment in Taiwan" on 14 September 2016, and representatives of the industry, government, professionals, physicians, pharmacists, patients, and legislators were invited to join the meeting. The opinions and advice from all sectors were collected to build strategies for preventing and treating hepatitis C.

By the time the new direct-acting antiviral agents for hepatitis C were launched in Taiwan, their prices were high, at more than New Taiwan dollars (NTD) 1 million for each treatment course. Therefore, the NHIA made every effort to negotiate with pharmaceutical firms for a price reduction. Meanwhile, the NHIA invited experts, scholars, and representatives of the medical providers, pharmaceutical firms, and patient groups to join a public hearing and then negotiated the budget in the National Health Insurance Committee (NHIC). Finally, the Ministry of Health and Welfare (MOHW) approved a 2017 budget of NTD 3.101 billion for the medications used for hepatitis C on 2 November 2016. Furthermore, the NHIA established a registry system for new, direct-acting antiviral agents for hepatitis C. The NHIA formally announced the "Implementation Plan of the Payment for New Direct-Acting Antiviral Agents for Hepatitis C in the National Health Insurance" and began to pay for the new direct-acting antiviral agents for hepatitis C on 24 January 2017.

As the MOHW is expecting that Taiwan could be a role model in the World Health Organization (WHO) and the World Health Assembly, the MOHW further proposed that Taiwan could achieve the WHO goal of eliminating hepatitis C by 2025. Therefore, the NHIA continues to receive higher budgets for hepatitis C medication in the NHIC and expands the reimbursement indications for the disease. Since 2019, patients infected with hepatitis C virus can be reimbursed for new direct-acting antiviral agents for hepatitis C without the limitation of being diagnosed with liver fibrosis.

According to National Hepatitis C Program Office estimates, there are about 405,000 hepatitis C patients in Taiwan. In the past, nearly 80,000 people have been successfully treated with interferon. To achieve the goal of eliminating hepatitis C, 250,000 people must receive new drug treatment. From 24 January 2017, to 31 December 2020, a total of 111,000 people have been treated with new drugs, and the treatment coverage rate is about 47.2%. We are almost halfway done in accomplishing the goal of eliminating hepatitis C in Taiwan by 2025.

Currently, we already have effective treatment for hepatitis B and C. The problem that we are facing in the future is to find people who don't know they are infected with hepatitis B and C. The MOHW has expanded the eligible age for subsidized adult preventive care service for hepatitis B and C screening, which is 45–79 years old, and the data can help the NHIA find patients.

Medical Device Reform Under National Health Insurance

Since the NHI first started operating 27 years ago, many efforts have been made to protect the health of all citizens. However, owing to the rapid development of new medical devices and the increasingly sophisticated functions and designs, the prices of devices are also rising. According to the statistics data, self-paid medical devices have increased annually to about 2750 items in 2020, and the total medical cost of self-paid medical devices is five times higher in 2020 than it was in 2014. People often question why the NHI does not cover new medical devices, and the other question is how to make the decision between NHI medical devices or self-paid ones.

As medical devices are highly professional products, the NHIA proactively cooperates with clinical professionals, takes clinical need as the main consideration, and promotes the reform of NHI medical devices to ensure the rights and interests of the public. After thoughtful and attentive discussion, there are three main problems:

1. The functions and types of self-paid medical devices are complicated, but which one is indispensable in the clinic?
2. How is coverage for new devices gradually expedited within the limited global budget?
3. Insufficient knowledge and information of medical devices leaves the public with limited choice.

Adding New Functional Categories of Medical Devices Based on Clinical Needs

Most people think that the items of the medical services and medicines paid for by the NHI should meet most people's "basic" medical needs. The NHI cannot cover all medical services, such as expensive new medical devices. If people want to use them, it is reasonable for them to pay for them themselves. Some people compare the NHI medical devices and special materials to domestic-made cars, people should pay more if they want to drive a Mercedes. However, this is not the way the NHI medical devices and special materials are classified. Different vehicles, such as sedans or SUVs, have different fuel tank sizes, equipment, and other settings. Choices have to be made according to the "function categories" and people's financial capabilities. Therefore, the medical devices under coverage of the NHI are based on the clinical needs of people. The "basic" medical needs are evolving with the times. Medical materials will be chosen for NHI coverage and classified based on the suggestions of medical associations and medical professionals. For the "clinical results" of the NHI medical devices, special materials, and self-paid medical devices, the comparison should be made on the basis of similar functional categories. In other words, it is more logical to compare medical materials with the same design purpose and similar clinical utilities, for example, comparing the nonlocking bone plate system and locking bone plate system used for fracture fixation.

Claims for Self-Paid Medical Devices Are Increasing

The NHIA has noticed that self-paid medical devices have gradually become the mainstream by analyzing the NHI claims data, while people continue to ask why does this belong to self-paid medical devices and why is that uncovered? Does this mean that the NHI medical devices and special materials have not met the basic clinical needs? Therefore, the NHIA checked all self-paid medical devices and found that nearly 60% are used for bone and neurological surgery and treatment. There are some self-paid medical devices that have similar functions to the NHI medical devices and special materials, but more than half of the claims are out-of-pockets, such as the locking plate system for fixing fractures (around 83%), intramedullary nails (around 58%), suture anchors for fixing soft tissues (around 60%), and artificial knee articular surface for treating degeneration (around 54%). It is even necessary for some of the self-paid medical devices to be covered, such as bone cement for spinal surgery, artificial cervical intervertebral discs that can maintain mobility for nonfusion surgery, and transcatheter replacement aortic valve sets required for new heart valve treatment techniques. Therefore, for these clinical indispensable devices with no similar NHI covering items provided, the NHIA, as the insurer of the NHI, has the responsibility to proactively strive for budget and cover medical devices to meet medical needs.

The NHIA faces these problems pragmatically and is promoting reforms progressively. We understand that medical devices are professional products, and clinicians are the frontline staff who understand the needs of patients the best. Therefore, we invite clinical experts from the medical associations, hospital representatives, and medical device license holders for communication and collect professional opinions on the clinical demand and how to set reasonable prices. At the same time, the NHIA has commissioned the Center for Drug Evaluation to establish a "value appraisal for progressing medical devices" to objectively evaluate the "clinical results" of the new medical devices, by collecting the evaluation results from clinical experts on the improvement in the treatment effect, patients' quality of life, medical cost efficacy, convenience in clinical operation, decrease in the adverse effects, and with the HTA report as a reference to the special medical materials expert consultation meeting. Then, the medical professionals will provide suggestions on whether to include the items in the NHI coverage or not.

Take transcatheter aortic valve implantation (TAVI), for example. It is a device for treating patients with severe aortic valve stenosis who cannot undergo surgery or for whom surgery is high risk. The NHIA used a value appraisal scheme to evaluate the new medical device, because it is a "new medical device with new medical technology" with no similar functional NHI medical devices and special materials. The NHIA has held three meetings to discuss with the cardiology-related specialty associations regarding this clinical "gap." Based on HTA reports and clinical professional recommendations, the proposal was discussed within the National Health Insurance Pharmaceutical Benefit and Reimbursement Scheme (PBRS) Joint Committee in November 2020, and was finally agreed to be covered by the NHI with full coverage from 1 February 2021. In addition, for artificial cervical intervertebral discs used in nonfusion spine surgery, the NHIA has also held seven meetings successively to communicate with relevant medical associations such as neurosurgery and orthopedics and will discuss reasonable payment as soon as possible. To increase clinical medical device choices for physicians, one HTA after another has been launched for self-paid medical devices, which are gradually replacing the NHI medical devices and special materials as the foundation of follow-up clinical professional discussions. The NHIA respects the professional opinions of the medical associations and works with the medical community to make decisions on incorporating new medical devices that truly meet clinical needs into NHI payments.

To increase the functional categories for new NHI medical devices, the NHIA has increased the budget for new medical devices annually, with NTD 522 million in 2017, NTD 610 million in 2018, NTD 585 million in 2019, NTD 400 million in 2020, and NTD 650 million in 2021. With collaboration with the medical community, NHIA hopes to gradually close the gap between clinical need and NHI medical device coverage.

Management of Balance-Billing of Medical Devices/Materials

As the medical industry develops and the population ages, the clinical demands for new medical devices increase. Building a sustainable NHI system under the limited NHI resources has always been the most important challenge for the NHIA. For this reason, second-generation NHI collects expensive medical devices that are more effective than the fully covered medical devices and special materials, and with unclear cost-effectiveness, as balance-billing materials. The NHI payment will cover part of the cost, whereas the rest will be paid by the patients. As a result, more new medical devices will be covered by the NHI payment, which increases the accessibility of new medical devices to patients.

In the past, the NHIA determined the payment of balance-billing medical devices based on the payment price of the most similar functional category item. However, it is difficult to find proper reference items owing to the rapid technology progressing or the balance-billing medical devices are too expensive to achieve the benefits of balance-billing. With the rapid development of the industry, most of the new medical devices have a short life cycle and clinical trials are not conducted before marketing. The industries often claim that the functional effect of the expensive devices is different from that of the NHI medical devices and special materials because of the patented design. However, the devices lack clinical evidence for the NHIA to determine reasonable payment. Therefore, the NHIA has promoted pragmatic reforms to incorporate the spirit of the "co-payment" into the payment method for NHI medical devices and special materials. To implement clinical evidence-based evaluation, the NHIA collects the true benefits of self-paid medical devices in clinical use and evaluates the difference between them and the NHI medical devices. The NHIA discusses the appropriate function/material classification with clinical professionals, and gradually includes clinically necessary self-paid medical devices into the NHI payments and pays reasonably based on clinical evidence. As a result, the NHI can take both finance and the richness of the NHI medical devices into consideration and implement the spirit of user charge at the same time.

To increase the types of the new medical devices for clinical application, the NHI strives to cooperate with the specialist medical associations to collect the items and pay at a reasonable balance-billing price. In the future, the NHIA will continue to follow the data on safety and efficacy to review the payment ratio, hoping to increase the clinical use of new medical devices, and clarify whether the self-paid medical devices are as effective as those claimed for by the public.

Information Transparency Enhances Shared Decision-Making Between Physicians and Patients

To help the public understand and search for the charging status of balance-billing medical devices in medical institutions and in order to increase information transparency, the NHIA established the "Price Comparison Platform of Medical Devices" in June 2014.. This platform is for NHI-contracted institutions to autonomously upload medical device charging information to facilitate accessibility to the public, and provides the public with a reference for choosing medical devices after comparison. The data are uploaded and self-checked by the contracted institutions. To improve the accessibility of the information, the NHIA carried out the following strategies:

1. Upgraded the app and Web function of the Price Comparison Platform of Medical Devices

   (a) To help the public inquiring about information, the NHIA gradually improved the function of the Price Comparison Platform of Medical Devices. The searching steps are as follows: Go to the Price Comparison Platform of Medical Devices, select the "Balance-Billing Item Charging Situation" tab, select "medical device" and "function/material classification," and then click the "Query" button to find out how the medical devices are charged in various NHI-contracted institutions. Advanced queries, such as specific counties and cities where the contracted institutions are located, contracted categories. and specific institutions, can also be searched in the query column; you can also search for the highest and lowest fees for each medical device item in the NHI-contracted institution (Fig. 9.7).

   (b) The Price Comparison Platform of Medical Devices can also be queried in the National Health Insurance Mobile Easy Access mobile application (NHI Express app). The search steps are as follows: open the app and go to the page of the Price Comparison Platform of Medical Devices. After reading the description page of the Balance-billing Medical Device, click "Go to Inquiry." Select "medical device" and "function/material classification" and click the "query" button to find out the charging information for the medical device in contracted institutions (Fig. 9.8).

2. Open data for the public
   The NHIA also published the Price Comparison Platform of Medical Devices data on the NHI Open Data website (https://data.nhi.gov.tw/Index.aspx) and structured the classification of functions and materials of the various balance-billing medical devices to facilitate accessibility to the user by direct application. In the future, the NHIA will continue to evolve the search function of the Price Comparison Platform of Medical Devices and optimize the website with the goal of being easier to "use," "search," and "compare" to improve the transparency and accessibility of information and enhance the communication between physicians and patients to achieve shared decision-making.

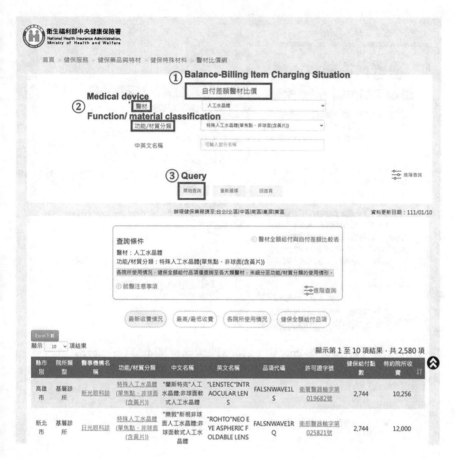

Fig. 9.7 Steps for usage of the Price Comparison Platform of Medical Devices web page

Conclusion

With the development of medical technology, personalized precision medicines have become mainstream cancer treatments. In response to accomplishing the goal of eliminating viral hepatitis by 2030 from the WHO, the coverage for hepatitis B and hepatitis C medications in the NHI has also been gradually expanding along with the latest clinical development. The NHIA makes efforts to safeguard the medical benefits and rights of the patients. Despite the rapid development of various medical technologies, medical expenses have also risen greatly, causing financial burdens on the NHI. The NHIA shoulders its responsibility and continues to work with the medical providers on good communication and focuses on seeking the balance between financial and clinical needs.

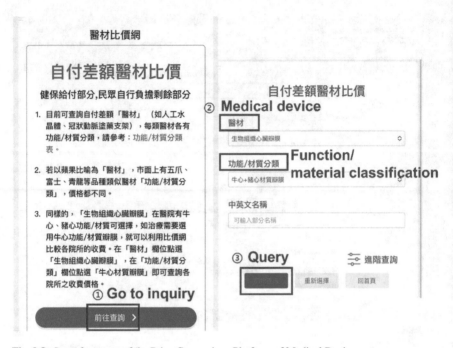

Fig. 9.8 Steps for usage of the Price Comparison Platform of Medical Devices app

Chapter 10
High-Value Medical Information and Quality Claims Review

Hsueh-Yung (Mary) Tai, Yu-Pin Chang, and Shwu-Huey Wu

Introduction

The medical expenses claimed by contracted medical institutions are mainly paid by the insurance premiums from those insured. The insurance premiums are limited resources and belong to public assets. To maximize the effectiveness of the premiums paid by those insured, and to make sure the medical resources are used appropriately on individuals, the National Health Insurance Administration (NHIA) aims to avoid unnecessary or inappropriate medical services and reimburse properly the providers who perform necessary and legitimate medical services.

Review Process of Medical Expense Claims

The NHIA complies with the National Health Insurance (NHI) Act and regulations, such as Article 62, "The insurer shall pay the medical expenses, according to the reviewed points, declared by contracted medical institutions." Article 63 "The insurer, in order to examine the item, quantity, and quality of the medical service of this insurance provided by the contracted medical institutions, shall appoint medical and pharmaceutical specialists who have clinical or relevant experience to conduct the review, which should be based on the approved payment; the review work should be assigned to the relevant professional agency or group. Review of the medical services in the preceding paragraph shall be done before, during, and after the matter; sampling or case analysis will be the methods used." Therefore, counseling and review are necessary.

H.-Y. (Mary) Tai (✉) · Y.-P. Chang · S.-H. Wu
National Health Insurance Administration, Ministry of Health and Welfare, Taipei, Taiwan
e-mail: marytai@nhi.gov.tw; A110413@nhi.gov.tw; shwu@nhi.gov.tw

© The Author(s) 2022
P.-C. Lee et al. (eds.), *Digital Health Care in Taiwan*,
https://doi.org/10.1007/978-3-031-05160-9_10

The Review Process

The regulations for medical claims processing, and review of the medical services of the NHI (hereinafter referred as the "Review") are authorized by the NHI Act to specify medical expense claims, procedures and schedules, and review of medical services (Fig. 10.1) as follows:

1. Pre-authorization review

    The NHIA could conduct pre-authorization reviews on the medical services, medical devices, and pharmaceuticals that are high risk, expensive, or easily abused in accordance with the fee schedule. If the contracted medical institution fails to make application of the medical services or report an item that is required for pre-authorization review, the NHIA can reject the reimbursement of the cases. The contracted medical institutions shall apply for pre-authorization reviews according to patient's conditions evaluated by physicians. The NHIA shall complete the pre-authorization review within 2 weeks and notify the contracted medical institutions. Furthermore, patients can also access the website of the NHIA regarding the progress of their applications (https://med.nhi.gov.tw/iwse0000/IWSE1010S02.aspx).

2. Review of medical claim

    The NHIA shall review the medical expense cases claimed by contracted medical institutions within 2 years, and these reviews include:

    (a) Procedure review

        The NHIA is striving to develop computerized case-by-case review (also known as automated medical order review) or file analysis. Some claimed

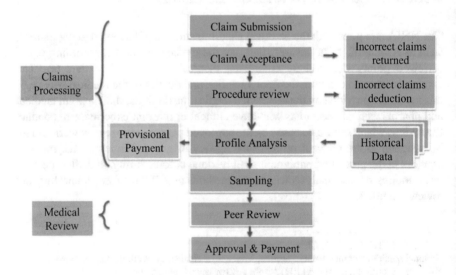

Fig. 10.1 Flow chart of medical claims processing and review

cases shall be ruled out from the procedure review, if those cases are non-compliant with regulations of the NHI—for instance, eligibility of the insured, scope of coverage, medical service items and fee schedules, pharmaceutical benefit, and reimbursement scheme.

(b) Professional review

Considering the capacity for professional review, there are two sampling methods: random sampling and purposive sampling. The random sampling means that medical expense claims will be randomly selected according to the sampling rate and the purposive sampling will be selected based on the results of the file analysis. The NHIA has implemented a global budget payment system, which was divided into four sectors, such as dental care, traditional Chinese medicine, primary-level Western medicine, and hospital care. According to the Act, the NHIA entrusted the Taiwan Hospital Association, Taiwan Medical Association, Taiwan Dental Association, and National Union of Chinese Medical Doctors' Association, R.O.C., with appointing medical and pharmaceutical specialists who have more than 5 years of teaching, clinical, or practical experience and have not violated the relevant health insurance laws and regulations, to conduct the professional review.

The medical services, medicines, and medical devices claimed by contracted medical institutions are subject to professional review, and if there are cases in which the medical services, drugs, and medical devices are inconsistent with the diagnosis of the disease or are unnecessary for examinations and hospitalization, the reimbursements will be reduced accordingly. For random sampling, the number of points will be scaled down based on the same proportion of sampling or the upper limit of scaled down negotiated by each sector of the global budget, whichever is lower, will be accepted; whereas for purposive sampling, the number of points will not be scaled down.

3. On-site review

The NHIA may inform the contracted medical institutions about the results of the file analysis from time to time, and designate personnel to conduct an on-site review of the manpower, medical facilities, and medical services provided by the medical providers. Thus, if the medical services were found to be improper or violated, consultation should be given for further improvement; also, the following measures could be taken according to the regulations, such as strengthening review frequency, reducing reimbursement, or conducting specific investigations under severe circumstances.

Relevant Regulations and References for the Review System

Regulations related to the reviews of medical expenses of the NHI include the "National Health Insurance Act," the "National Health Insurance Medical Service Payment Items and Fee Schedule," the "National Health Insurance Drug Dispensing Items and Fee Schedule," and the "National Health Insurance Medical Claim

Review Notices," etc.. All laws and regulations are published on the website of the NHIA Global Information Network.

Administrative Remedy Mechanism for Contracted Medical Institutions

There are three levels of administrative remedy for the NHI medical claims: preliminary review, appeal review, and dispute review. Although the contracted medical institution submits the medical claims, from the 1st of the month after the contracted medical institution provides medical services, it has been entering the NHIA's preliminary review. If the contracted medical institution finds the determination of the preliminary review unacceptable, it may file a petition stating the reasons and accompanied by documentary evidence and request for an appeal review. The abovementioned petition shall be made within 60 days from the date of arrival of the notification from the NHIA. If the insured person or the contracted medical institution remains unconvinced of the decision of the appeal review, they can submit a dispute review to the National Health Insurance Dispute Mediation Committee (another independent unit) of the Ministry of Health and Welfare (MOHW, see Fig. 10.2). The procedures of the dispute review application, the timeline of the application period, and the attached documents can be found on the website of the National Health Insurance Dispute Mediation Committee (https://dep.mohw.gov.tw/NHIDSB/lp-1607-117.html).

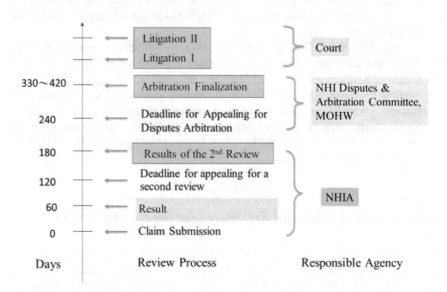

Fig. 10.2 Medical claim, review, and appeal process

Strengthening Front-End Claims Management

For the sustainable development of the NHI system, the NHIA continues to conduct medical expense review operations under the premise of respecting the medical profession. It is used to guide contracted medical institutions to provide medical services in accordance with the payment regulations, avoid detractions from the compensation of necessary medical services, and return the limited resources of the NHI to reasonable payment for conscientious medical personnel. The real purpose of the review is to implement the regulations, not to deduct the payment. Therefore, for the more transparent review information, the NHIA plans to proactively remind the contracted medical institutions about the management priorities before the medical expenses claimed.

Progress the Review Operation to Avoid Deprivatizing Disputes

Owing to the high level of medical accessibility in Taiwan, the average number of medical visits per person per year is currently 15, about 370 million claims are made in a year, and it is impossible to conduct professional reviews of all claims while considering manpower and administrative costs. Through big data analysis, the NHIA submits sample medical records to medical peers for professional review, and the sample's medical expense reduction rate is taken as the reduction rate of the population.

However, the operations of professional peer reviews had caused considerable controversy in the past. There were even rumors that the reviews were carried out by part-time workers, or the deletion was determined randomly by electric fans. The results of the deletion also triggered protests by physicians or complaints through social media platforms. One of the main reasons for such controversial issues was that the passive review mechanism did not provide full disclosure to medical institutions to acknowledge the management priorities, which led to a sense of deprivation of medical personnel who worked hard in health care.

To cope with controversies from the old style reviews in the past, the NHIA not only improves the review strategies and methods continuously, but also executes a more proactive and transparent method to allow contracted medical institutions to manage together. Meanwhile, the NHIA clearly reminds the contracted medical institutions that their main responsibility is to set management priorities on taking care of patients, so as to strengthen the institutional management mechanism.

Since 2018, the NHIA has assembled big data profiles and consultations of crucial abnormal cases from medical expertise to feedback to medical institutions as references to facilitate their self-improvement. For example, the case "Appropriateness of reprocessing after total hysterectomy" concerned the patient who received a total hysterectomy, if subsequent uterine-related treatment was performed, there was a certain degree of unreasonableness, and it was necessary to

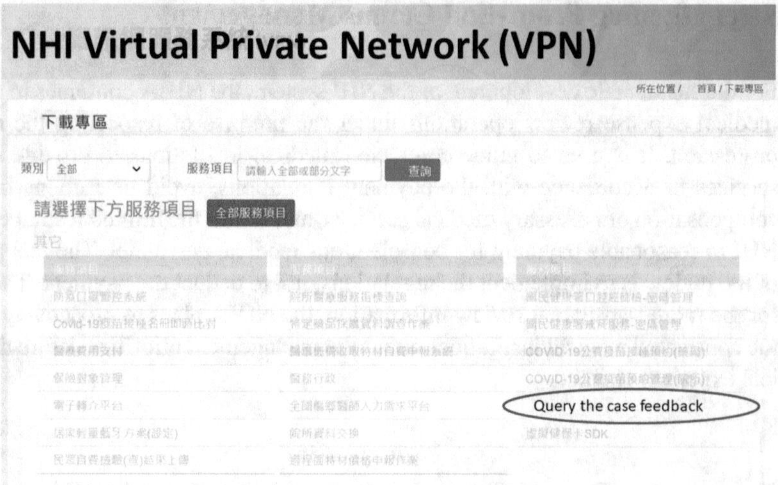

圖片來源：健保署健保資訊網服務系統(https://medvpn.nhi.gov.tw/iwse0000/IWSE0030S01.aspx)

Fig. 10.3. Query the case feedback

check how appropriate it was. In another case, "Management of abnormal declaration of new oral drug for hepatitis C" (Fig. 10.3), according to Point 6 of Item 9 of the "Implementation Plan of the Payment for New Oral Drugs for Hepatitis C in the NHI (revised on 21 September 2020)," which was announced by the NHIA, each case can only have one treatment combination and the payment is limited in one treatment course. However, according to statistics, from January 2017 to December 2018 in all hospitals, it was found that there were abnormal situations such as repeated treatment combinations, and the number of medical claims exceeded the upper limit of the course. The total number of relative value unit (RVUs) deducted was 43 million. The NHIA has also conducted automated medical reviews to prevent the contracted medical institutions from claiming in the wrong way.

Pre-Inspection of Medical Expense Claims

Many clinicians claim that most of the deletions are caused by the unfamiliarity of the payment regulations; therefore, the NHIA builds an inspection program before the review, such as payment regulations being limited to specific payment items that must be implemented for specific patients' age, gender, or physician's specialty qualifications. The relevant payment items and prescribed procedures have been built for pre-inspection by contracted medical institutions before uploading the claims, so as to reduce the subsequent deletions. For instance, "artificial electronic ear" is limited to patients aged under 18, the use of patients over 18 years old is not in compliance with the regulations. In addition, the medical service "68040B/

Transcatheter Aortic Valve Replacement" must be performed by a cardiologist and a cardiac surgery specialist in a joint operation. Therefore, it is not in compliance with the requirements if physicians who do not have the front-listed specialist quali-fications perform the operation.

Implementation of Institutional Self-Management

The NHIA upholds the spirit of cooperating with institutions, to cope with past pas-sive review mechanisms, and to provide a more transparent and active reminder mechanism, so that the contracted medical institutions can access the management priorities and merge them into the institutional self-management. Assembling of resources and undergoing joint management programs not only reduce the increas-ing number of disputes from the reviews but also simplifies the follow-up adminis-trative tasks, such as reclama, dispute mediation, and others, to jointly create new value for the NHI.

Integrating Examination and Test Results and Medical Claims Uploaded by Contracted Institutions

To enable medical professionals to quickly query the medical information of patients in different medical institutions for diagnosis and treatment when people are seek-ing medical care and improve patient safety and efficiency of medical care, the NHIA actively assists in increasing the network bandwidth of contracted medical institutions and promotes the "National Health Insurance Incentive Plan of Medical Institutions Querying Patients' Medical Information in Real Time" (hereinafter referred to as "Plan of Querying in Real Time") to speed up the information transfer. This plan not only allows medical institutions to upload examination and test results in real time and query patients' medical information when people are seeking medi-cal care but also assists in finding abnormalities by artificial intelligence (AI) review. In addition, people can query medical information through the National Health Insurance Mobile Easy Access mobile application (NHI Express app) to strengthen self-health management.

Strengthening the Network Infrastructure and Coverage Rate

The first key to speeding up data flow is the network infrastructure. In the past, most of the primary-level clinics submitted the claim through an asymmetric digital sub-scriber line to the NHI virtual private network (VPN), which was slow and poor in quality. Therefore, the NHIA strove for subsidies to build a fiber-optic network and continued to coordinate preferential rental plans with telecommunication operators. Based on the principle of encouragement and gradual implementation, the NHIA has subsidized the monthly rental fees for the leased-line network for medical institutions since 2014. However, the subsidy method is to subsidize 50% of the network expenses first, and then the remaining 50% will be subsidized after the medical institution reaches the target set by the NHIA. Medical institutions have deployed fiber-optic networks through this program, and the fiber-optic network deployment rate of Western medical institutions has increased from 37% in 2015 to 94% in February 2021 (Table. 10.1).

Improving the Integrity of Real-Time Uploaded Data

After the promotion of the My Health Bank System in 2014, people generally expressed their willingness to access their examination and test results to facilitate self-care for health, and the NHIA also followed this opinion to develop the Plan of Querying in Real Time. In 2015, the examination and test results and discharge summary was added; in 2016, the implant of artificial joints data were added; in 2017, the referral data were added, and the monthly rental fees for the mobile network were subsidized to facilitate the data transmission and query, whereas medical institutions provided home care services outside the hospital or provided medical services in the underserved and remote areas; in 2018, medical image data were added, such as computed tomography (CT), MRI, X-rays, and clinical microscopy, and the subsidies for increasing network bandwidth in hospitals were expanded to accelerate transmission of medical image data; from 2019 to 2020, the uploaded items were added continuously, and there were a total of 689 rewarded upload items (642 kinds of examination and test results, 47 kinds of medical images) as of February 2021; in 2020, the claimed medical orders of rewarded upload items accounted for more than 80% of all examinations and tests, which means the uploaded data of examinations and tests have become more complete.

Table. 10.1 Virtual private network bandwidth upgrade from an asymmetric digital subscriber line to optical fiber

	2015 (%)	2016 (%)	2017 (%)	2018 (%)	2019 (%)	2020 (%)
Medical center	100	100	100	100	100	100
Regional hospital	100	100	100	100	100	100
District hospital	80	89	93	98	99	100
Clinic	25	37	43	76	94	95
Chinese medicine clinic	17	44	59	72	91	95
Dental clinic	21	39	46	64	85	90
Pharmacy	26	35	40	49	82	91
Others	2	3	7	15	76	89

Medical Information Is Fully Uploaded in Real Time

As of December 2020, a total of 27,353 medical institutions were participating in the Plan of Querying in Real Time (participation rate 93%), including 470 hospitals (participation rate 100%) and 19,769 clinics (participation rate 94%); since the Plan of Querying in Real Time was launched in 2015, there have been 3.4 billion examinations and test results and 68.07 million medical images uploaded by medical institutions as of December 2020; the hospital upload rate of examinations, test results, and medical images in 24 h also increased year by year, and exceeded 80% by 2020 (Figs. 10.4 and 10.5).

Strengthening the Uploading of Medical Information and the Integration of Claims for Reimbursement

In the current review practice, fraudulence has been found in that some hospitals submitted a claim without providing corresponding medical services or duplicated claims. According to the claims data of medical examinations, tests, and medical images combined with the uploaded examination and test results and medical images, it was found that the upload rate of clinics was low (Tables 10.2, 10.3 and Figs. 10.6, 10.7, 10.8, and 10.9).

Broadly speaking, the complete claims data submitted to the NHIA by medical institutions should include the claim for reimbursement and the implementation data of providing medical services, such as results and reports of examinations and test and medical images (including reports). To meet the principles of claiming according to the medical services actually provided, it is necessary to upload the relevant report in the medical process. The NHIA will first review the cases that have been claimed, but the examination and test results have not been uploaded to

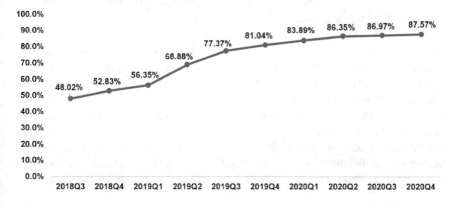

Fig. 10.4 Trend of real-time upload rate of examination and test results (2018Q3–2020Q4)

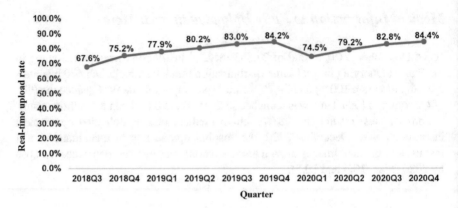

Fig. 10.5 Trend of real-time upload rate of medical images (2018Q3–2020Q4)

Table 10.2 Implementation status of plan of querying in real time in 2020—examination and test results

	Claim records (cases)	Uploaded records (cases)	Upload rate (cases) (%)	RVUs of claim records (RVUs)	RVUs of uploaded records (RVUs)	RVUs without uploaded records (RVUs)
Hospitals	291 million	267 million	**91.9**	49.4 billion	37.5 billion	**11.8 billion**
Clinics	26.5 million	5.24 million	**19.7**	5.1 billion	420 million	**4.6 billion**

Table 10.3 Implementation status of plan of querying in real time in 2020—medical images

	Claim records (cases)	Uploaded records (cases)	Upload rate (cases) (%)	RVUs of claim records (RVUs)	RVUs of uploaded records (RVUs)	Upload rate (RVUs) (%)
Hospitals	39.49 million	31.80 million	**80.5**	33.6 billion	29.2 billion	**86.9**
Clinics	6.09 million	16,000	**0.3**	2.5 billion	60 million	**2.4**

understand in depth whether there is any fraudulence that medical institutions submitted the claim to the NHIA without providing corresponding medical services.

However, medical institutions now upload the medical information following the Plan of Querying in Real Time, which is only an incentive plan. To achieve the goal of fully uploading, the NHIA reviews laws and payment regulations of examinations and tests of the National Health Insurance, such as "Regulations Governing the Production and Issuance of the NHI Card and Data Storage," to make laws and regulations more comprehensive. Eventually, provided that medical services correspond with the claims data, the uploaded data will also correspond to the claims data.

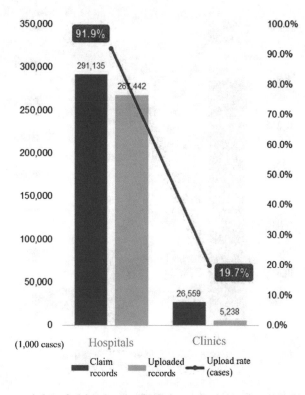

Fig. 10.6 Case statistics of claimed and uploaded examination and test results in the Plan of Querying in Real Time in 2020

Strengthening the Connection Between the Contracted Institution Hospital Information System and the National Health Insurance Information System—Usage of the Medical Visit Identifier and Timely Upload Improves Data Accuracy

To comply with the trend toward cloud services and big data applications, the NHIA integrates the monthly medical claims data, the daily uploaded medical visit data of the NHI card, and others to establish a "people-centered" database. In 2013, the "NHI PharmaCloud System" was built, and its scope was expanded in 2015 to become the "National Health Insurance MediCloud System (NHI MediCloud System)." Since 2017, the function of uploading and sharing medical images, such as CT and MRI, was added. The system could be accessed online by clinicians to understand the patient's medical history as a basis for prescribing drugs or inspections. In addition to safeguarding medication safety for patients, it can also save unnecessary costs of examinations and tests. The NHI MediCloud System and the Hospital Information System (HIS) are linked closely through the NHI Application Programming Interfaces (APIs) and a VPN. The contracted medical institutions and

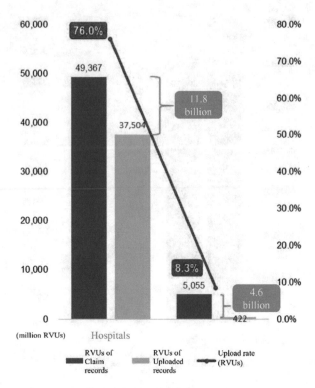

Fig. 10.7 Relative value unit statistics of claimed and uploaded examination and test results in the Plan of Querying in Real Time in 2020

the data on the NHI MediCloud System are promptly connected, and the information is shared across institutions. The interaction between the two is thus more closely linked.

However, there are still the following issues that may affect the effectiveness of the NHI Big Data applications in practice. According to Article 10 of the "Regulations Governing the Production and Issuance of the National Health Insurance IC Card and Data Storage": the contracted medical institutions shall upload the medical records within 24 h after they have been registered on the NHI IC cards to the insurer for future reference. Most institutions upload batches daily, but some do not know how to correct or write off prescriptions after uploading the medical records. As a result, the information on the NHI MediCloud System might be incorrect, or people might find abnormal medical records through the My Health Bank System. Moreover, the information systems of the NHI such as the NHI MediCloud System, e-Referral Platform, and the NHI Express App have to connect the medical service items (such as examinations and tests, drug dispensing, medical images) received by the public at the time of medical treatment, but some data cannot be connected owing to the inconsistency of the primary key value. Other related businesses in the NHIA, such as comparing the medical claims data between the clinic that released

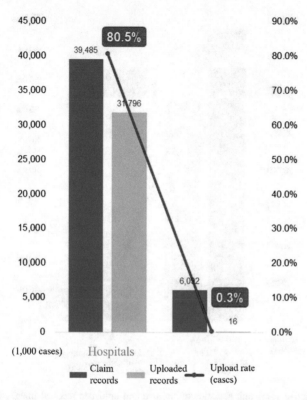

Fig. 10.8 Case statistics of claimed and uploaded medical images in the Plan of Querying in Real Time in 2020

the prescription and the dispensing pharmacy, or other statistical analysis applications on personal medical visits, may also encounter the above situation, resulting in a decrease in data accuracy. In addition, if the insured person reissues a prescription at the institution owing to a change in medical condition or claims that the prescription is lost, and then holds the original prescription (or holds the printed prescription) to the pharmacy for repeated dispensing, the pharmacy cannot verify from the NHI MediCloud System regardless of whether or not the prescription has been canceled (prescription validity).

To improve the connection with the information of the institution's HIS and the quality and safety of medical care for people, the NHIA has developed enhanced measures for the timeliness and accuracy of medical data. The instructions are as follows:

1. Functional improvements of the information system for the NHIA

   (a) Timeliness: the relevant data flow and system structure have been adjusted to receive the medical visit data of the NHI IC card. The system adopts

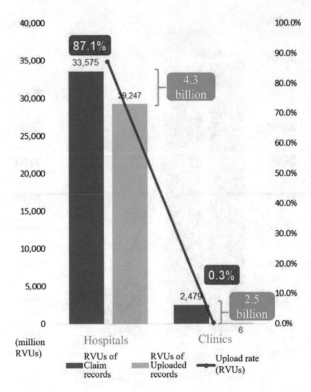

Fig. 10.9 Relative value unit statistics of claimed and uploaded medical images in the Plan of Querying in Real Time in 2020

parallel technology to do data checking, and the checked data will be synchronized to the NHI MediCloud System timely.

(b) Accuracy: the NHIA developed the correcting operation for the medical visit data of the NHI IC card, in response to the situations that contacted the NHIA regional division for correcting the uploaded data, to improve the accuracy of the sharing information such as the My Health Bank System or the NHI MediCloud System.

(c) Establishing the mechanism of the "medical visit identifier": to facilitate the concatenation of individual medical information and confirm the validity of prescriptions.

(d) Planning to build a timely uploading mechanism of the NHI IC card medical visit data for canceled prescriptions: when pharmacies are dispensing, they can check whether or not the prescriptions have been canceled on the NHI MediCloud System.

2. The strengthening measures planned for the contracted institutions

(a) The clinics provide a timely upload of medical treatment information: the NHIA coaches the institutions to upload the medical information to the

NHIA within 6–8 h after providing medical services, speeding up the data flow.

(b) Simplify the correction operation of the uploaded NHI IC card medical visit data: for data with the same primary key value, adjust the process to improve the accuracy of the NHI MediCloud System data.

(c) Establish a medical visit-identified mechanism (Fig. 10.10):

  (i) Every time people seek medical care, the HIS of the institution contacts the NHIA's card reader control software for a medical visit identifier generated by a special calculation function.

 (ii) The "medical visit identifier" is a unique 20-digit code consisting of the institution code, time code, and personal ID for an individual medical visit. It can be printed as a bar code if necessary so that a bar code scanner can acquire the medical information instead of manual input.

(iii) After people receive medical services, the medical visit identifier with the combination of the medical visit data of the NHI IC card and the medical claim data is uploaded to the NHIA to improve the accuracy of subsequent data concatenation.

(d) The timely upload and cancelation of the prescription mechanism for the institutions: upload the contents of the prescription with the medical visit data of the NHI card for the pharmacy to confirm the prescription validity. If a prescription is delivered during the medical visit, the medical visit data of the NHI card must be uploaded within a certain period for the pharmacy to query on the NHI MediCloud System to check whether the prescription can be dispensed (Fig. 10.11).

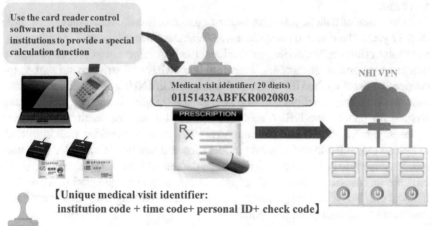

Use the card reader control software at the medical institutions to provide a special calculation function

Medical visit identifier(20 digits)
01151432ABFKR0020803

PRESCRIPTION

NHI VPN

【Unique medical visit identifier:
institution code + time code+ personal ID+ check code】

5 digits(medical institution abbreviation code)+ 7 digits(year, month, day, hour and minute abbreviation code)+ 7 digits(ID abbreviation code)+ 1 digit(check code)

Fig. 10.10 The principle of the medical visit identifier production system and the providing method

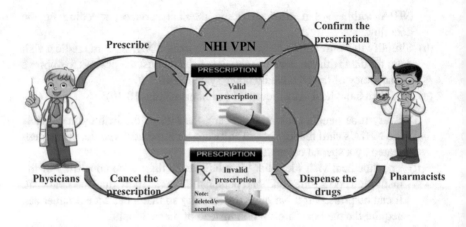

Fig. 10.11 Both the prescribing site and the dispensing site confirm the validity of the prescription by the "medical visit identifier"

Conclusion

Under the government's facilitation of the Digital Nation and Innovative Economic Development Program, emerging technologies are continuously transforming the healthcare industry. The NHI Big Data is an important national asset supporting the business advancement of the NHI, health and medical management decisions, and the value-added applications in the biomedical industry with the support of legislation.

"The value of data begins with integrity and precision." Accumulated for more than 27 years, the rich and comprehensive database of the NHI consists of the long-term joint efforts of the NHIA, institutions, medical information and communication vendors, and other partners. Therefore, the NHIA will strive to strengthen the connection between the HIS of the institutions and the NHI information to improve data accuracy and timeliness, to enhance its applicability in the My Health Bank System for people, the NHI MediCloud System for medical institutions, and AI reviews. The NHIA will also continue to provide medical facilities with incentives to upload examination and test data in real time and bundle the uploaded data with reimbursement to secure the integrity of the dataset. It is hoped that, utilized properly, the information system will help the NHIA to achieve the goal of increasing medical efficiency, reducing medical expenditure, developing smart health care, and improving the health of all residents.

Chapter 11
Applications of Big Data and Artificial Intelligence

Hsueh-Yung (Mary) Tai

Introduction

In 2019, the National Health Insurance Administration (NHIA) conducted approximately 2.53 million cases of medical claim reviews and 430,000 cases of pre-authorization reviews. However, contracted medical institutions invested countless hours of labor and sheets of paper in photocopying medical charts, and the cost of postal fees in mailing them to the NHIA if they choose to submit hard copies for claim reviews. Nevertheless, the reviewing physicians have to acknowledge profound information, such as relevant regulations and/or rules, fee schedules, and clinical guidelines to distinguish the severity of cases and the need for medications. The items mentioned above are all challenges to the reviewers. Therefore, the NHIA initiated and introduced the use of big data to set up several digital claim reviewing tools and train artificial intelligence (AI) to improve reviewing efficacy. By referring to data profiles, the NHIA can detect abnormal or unusual claims and reduce medical waste with efficiency.

Application of Big Data

To ensure the sustainable operation of the National Health Insurance (NHI) system and to conduct the proper use of limited resources efficiently, the NHIA set up a big data management model for executing precise reviews. A screening platform (Fig. 11.1) was established in 2013 to target claims that are suspected of consuming

H.-Y. (Mary) Tai (✉)
National Health Insurance Administration, Ministry of Health and Welfare, Taipei, Taiwan
e-mail: marytai@nhi.gov.tw

© The Author(s) 2022
P.-C. Lee et al. (eds.), *Digital Health Care in Taiwan*,
https://doi.org/10.1007/978-3-031-05160-9_11

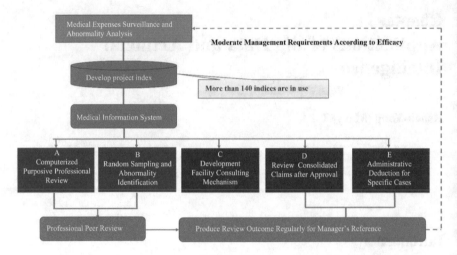

Fig. 11.1 Central Intelligence System Abnormal or unusual claim screening platform

medical resources abnormally. Abnormal or unusual claims are screened out of the platform automatically and flagged as peer review targets, and then sent for the review procedure. Alert messages were sent to the NHIA to facilitate the targeting of medical records and have compliance with NHI regulations. The prompt monitoring improves the overall review effectiveness. This system has nearly 140 screening indicators in five main domains, i.e., outpatient and inpatient services, drugs, specific diagnosis and treatments, and target cases for guiding purposes. It is estimated that from 2017 to the third quarter of 2020, a total of 700 million relative value units (RVUs) were deducted after professional peer reviews and reallocated back to the global budget to support the value of RVUs.

Big Data Analysis as the Most Useful Tool

In recent years, under the premise of professional autonomy, the NHIA has also actively adopted data analysis as the main tool for claim review. Various statistical data analysis was used to detect abnormal healthcare-seeking behavior, medical institution diagnosis, treatment types, and medical expense claims. Multiple measures are implemented to carry out key management focuses.

Reduce Duplicated Medications

The NHIA has implemented outpatient duplicated medication management strategies for specific drugs since July 2015 and expanded the drug management project in October 2017, from six categories to 12. In 2019, the management scope was

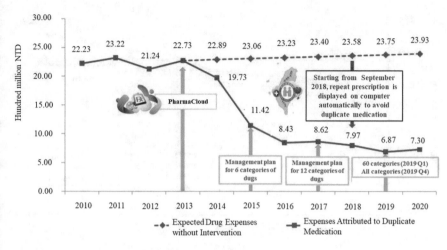

Fig. 11.2 Outcome of duplicated medication reduction

expanded from 12 to 60 categories, covering approximately 70% of the medical insurance's outpatient drug items. From October 2019, the management was further expanded to all-oral drugs in outpatient clinics. It is hoped that waste of medication can be prevented through the joint efforts of all contracted medical facilities, in the process of either prescription or dispensing. Based on the average annual growth rate, it is estimated that from 2014 to 2020, nearly 9.35 billion RVUs in repeated drug expenditure were saved (Fig. 11.2).

Avoid Unnecessary Medical Examinations and Tests

To reduce unnecessary medical expenses, the NHIA proactively applies information technology and big data analysis methods to aggregate patients' medical information in different hospitals. In this way, doctors can refer to the quick reminder on drug or exam duplication provided on the National Health Insurance MediCloud System (NHI MediCloud System) for treatment and diagnosis. In addition, since July 2017, contracted medical institutions or physicians who have higher execution and re-execution rates for 20 categories of examination than their peers would receive feedback to encourage self-management. Furthermore, physicians who order computed tomography (CT) or magnetic resonance imaging (MRI) without checking outpatient images and test results uploaded to the NHI MediCloud System by other facilities within 28 days are subject to counseling and are guided. From 2018 to 2020, the cost of repeated examinations and tests for 44 types in outpatient clinics was reduced by approximately 1 billion RVUs (Fig. 11.3).

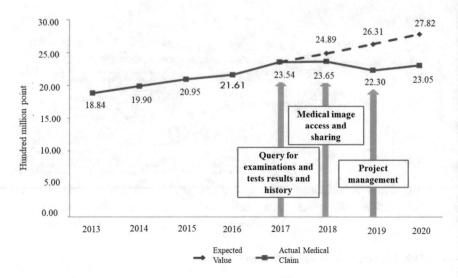

Fig. 11.3 Outcome of unnecessary tests and examination reduction

1. Develop monitoring platforms for the medical utilization of specific diagnosis and treatment types

   (a) Customized hemophilia medical history

      To allow hemophilia patients to obtain individualized and appropriate treatment, the NHIA established a hemophilia case management system in 2020 to thoroughly record each patient's disease type, severity, each bleeding situation, and dose and timing of coagulation factor injections that were brought home, and the results of regular medical evaluations. This repository of documents includes the treatment histories of hemophilia patients and enhances their care continuity when they switch treatment facilities. Because there is no need to worry about the interruption of the treatment record, each patient's treatment can be sustainable, undergoing monitoring and evaluation for its appropriateness and compliance with the NHI drug benefits regulations to ensure reasonable utilization of medical resources.

   (b) Medical utilization management for nursing home residents

      Since 2012, the NHIA has been developing a decision-making support system, which regularly collects medical utilization data from residents in nursing homes, guided targets, and screening indicators through systematic analysis. For health facilities that deliver excessive medical services, the NHIA further review the appropriateness of their medical services and provide professional consultation with the medical institutions for modification, hoping to maintain the quality of medical care and avoid wastage of medical resources.

Digitalization of Review Tools

Nowadays, information technology is advancing at lightning speed, and it is necessary for the NHIA to keep pace with the developments and improvements of information technologies to make medical claim review procedures more efficient.

Making Good Use of Technology to Simplify the Process

The "Paper-Based Medical Record Alternative Professional Review Program" was launched to encourage contracted medical institutions to convert their hard copies into electronic files and submit them via a virtual private network (VPN) online. This program is aimed at saving expenditure on human resources, equipment, consumables, and storage space that traditional paper medical record submission requires, improve the quality of materials submitted for review, and effectively save energy and reduce paper consumption.

In recent years, the NHIA has vigorously promoted the digital transformation of reviews, and more than 90% of pre-authorization review cases have submitted claims online. The levels of digitalization for medical reimbursement claims are related to the information capabilities of the hospital. Not surprisingly, medical centers and regional hospitals have the highest level of digitalization. Accumulatively more than 3000 hospitals and clinics have participated in digital transformation, indicating the popularity of online submission for review documents.

Continuing the successful experience of promoting online submission for reviews, the NHIA introduced more user-friendly tools to crosscheck the tremendous amount of reimbursement claim data, review materials, and reference documents to accurately display important review information promptly. Here are some important attributes of the upgraded "Intelligent Professional Review System":

1. Automatic comparison of medical records for preliminary review and appeal review

    Because the size of documents submitted for reviews by hospitals is tremendously large, the types of files vary as well. Therefore, considerable efforts must be made by the reviewing physicians to go over the medical records. Soon after the introduction of IT to integrate PDF files for the medical records submitted for reviews, the system then processed bookmarks for queries and automatically flagging the differences. It helps the reviewing physicians to be able to quickly grasp the supplements of the hospital and key points of the appeal review.

2. Smart linkage to regulations

    Linkage between each medical order to the NHI regulations and review key points was installed; therefore, the reviewing physicians can check the latest and/ or updated provisions by all means.

Monthly Medical Visit Statistics by Department (growth rate)

Department	Case no.	Prescription day	Diagnosis	Pharmaceutical Services	Drug	Treatment	Total Points	Points Claimed	Co-payment	Medical fee per case	Treatment fee per case	Daily drug fee	Prescription day
		Fee for									Average		
Cardiovascular Surgery	-6.92%	0%	-0.2%	-7.23%	8.07%	3.29%	5.17%	5.70%	-3.93%	13.01%	11.03%	17.52%	-1.20%

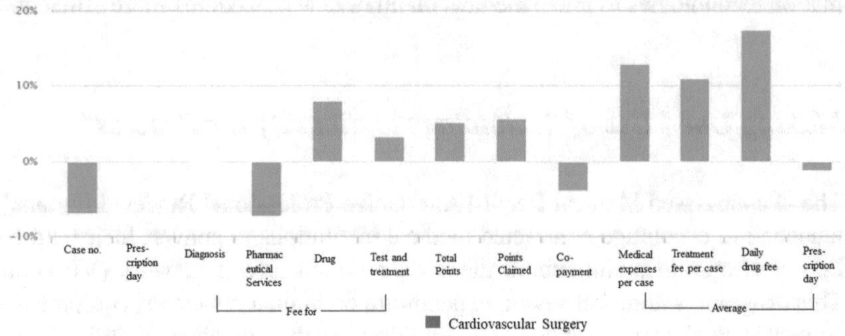

Fig. 11.4 Breakdown of medical expenses by specialties

3. Integration of Medical Records and Visualization of Key Reviewing Points (Fig. 11.4)

   The platform actively compiles patients' medical records and verifies whether they meet the NHI regulations. Key reviewing points are displayed as charts or tables so that the reviewing physician can extract information more intuitively.

4. Mistake proofing reminder and individualized setting: considering that reviewing physicians are very busy during the review process, the platform is designed with various mistake-proof mechanisms that detect improper operations, real-time reminders, and individualized settings such as frequently used phrases, modifiable window size, etc., to create a user-friendly intelligent review system

Engage Medical Communities in a Collaborative Environment by Precise Management and Message Feedback

The traditional table format has been abandoned by the NHIA; an interactive interface and a visualized platform were introduced to optimize the appearance of screening indicators and review results, which assists colleagues of the NHIA and hospital administrators to quickly identify abnormal or unusual medical claims. An interactive management model, originally designed for internal use, has been shared with the medical community through the NHI VPN information network system. The NHIA plans to overhaul the professional review process, which includes sampling, submission for review, special review, and result feedback. This gradually carries out the digitalized review process and improves the efficiency of the health insurance system together with the medical industry and may cause the quality management of medical resources.

Application of Artificial Intelligence Facilitates Enhanced Review Efficiency

The NHI database has abundant structured and unstructured data. It is estimated that in 2019, there were about 370 million entries of structured data, mostly medical claims data from outpatient clinics, and about 12.3 billion entries of unstructured data; test, and examination results and images constitute the majority. However, without a proper process or manipulation, the application of unstructured data is merely limited, time consuming, and labor intensive.

In 2019, there were approximately 2.53 million medical claims and 430,000 pre-authorization review cases. On average, each reviewing physician needs to review more than 100 cases at each session. In addition to the heavy load of reviewing cases, NHI regulations are quite diverse and complicated, and it is not easy for reviewing physicians to commence manual comparison among different medical records or materials, or relevant review regulations. Thus, a logical sampling method was adopted by the NHIA in 2019 to help reviewers to empower capabilities on professional reviews.

Moreover, the agency facilitated its database and reduced the workloads of professional reviews by integrating the results of big data analysis in the review system, which helps doctors to focus on the key points of reviews and accurately process the review mechanisms through intelligent IT systems.

Automatic Intelligent Review System Prompts in the Professional Review System

To consolidate all the information required for professional reviews and reduce the manual work of physicians, the results of big data analysis have been installed into the NHI professional review system so that various review key points, such as statistics on medical utilization, histories of claim reduction, and alert messages, will display automatically and promptly on the reviewing physician's screen. Another example is the pre-authorization review cases. If there are violations such as using oncological immunotherapy drugs in combination with target drugs, suggestions of nonsuitable medication for patients on rheumatoid arthritis immune drugs, history of traditional anti-rheumatic drugs, and test results found by the system, then the results of findings and/or alert messages will be displayed automatically to help reviewing physicians to quickly grasp the key points of the case, which greatly simplifies manual procedures for professional reviews and payment regulation comparisons.

Artificial Intelligence-Assisted Precision Review

The NHIA wisely uses big data and AI technology for assistance with combining structured claim data, unstructured examination results, and images to develop intelligence-assisted precision inspection mechanisms (Fig. 11.5), such as "image and report quality monitoring" and "duplicated or similar image detection."

1. Monitoring of image or report quality before claims are uploaded

The NHIA encourages contracted medical institutions to upload medical images and unstructured texts of examination results promptly. A total of 12.3 billion pieces of data were uploaded in 2019; however, there were difficulties in reviewing or analyzing, owing to unstructured, incomplete, or incorrect data.

To cope with the huge and complex amount of uploaded data and enhance the application value of big data, the NHIA established a quality monitoring system for uploaded claims data, including medical images, CT and MRI examination text reports, and hepatitis C and kidney function test results. In this way, the NHIA can use big data analysis to monitor the quality of the data uploaded by contracted medical institutions. For example, the system detects whether images uploaded are consistent with their medical orders, validates whether the content of the image text reports contain image findings or assumptions, and checks whether the data uploaded conform to the report format, etc.

Monitoring results as feedback can be sent to medical institutions in a timely manner to assist with the improvement of data quality and consequently enhance the application values of the health insurance database and the efficiency of cloud data sharing.

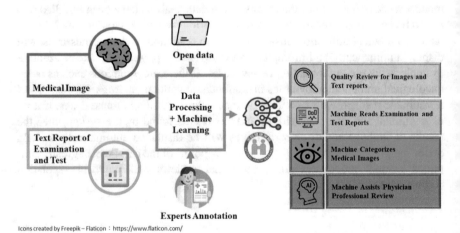

Icons created by Freepik – Flaticon : https://www.flaticon.com/

Fig. 11.5 Artificial intelligence-assisted precision review

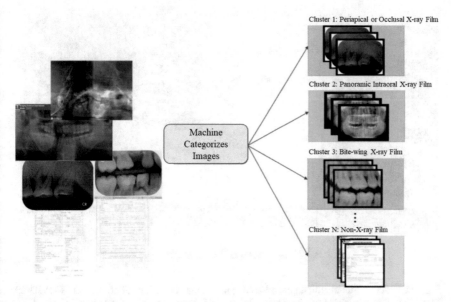

Fig. 11.6 The concept of grouping for a similar image detection tool. (Source: NHI Data Warehouse)

2. Detection of duplicate or similar images submitted for review

The NHIA has discovered some sporadic cases from contracted medical institutions that were suspected of submitting identical images as review materials for different cases. To reduce physicians' burden of reviewing more than 70,000 dental and cataract imaging review cases per month, an AI technology reviewing tool was developed to automatically detect duplicate dental and cataract images (Fig. 11.6). This tool can search through 1000 images in 5 s and complete 1000 pairs of dental and cataract image similarity detections in 6 min, assisting review for physicians in interpreting duplicates or very similar images without difficulty.

The application of AI technology replaces the ineffective labor-intensive comparison of medical images when detecting repetition and significantly improves the precision and effectiveness of the image review process.

Applying Artificial Intelligence Technology to Epidemic Prevention

1. Transformation of the review process for rheumatoid arthritis immunization drugs

As more than 30,000 cases of rheumatoid arthritis immunization drugs are reviewed each year, the NHIA gives it a high priority in revising the professional review process. Computerized comparisons between self-inspected documents submitted by contracted medical institutions and predictions generated by AI

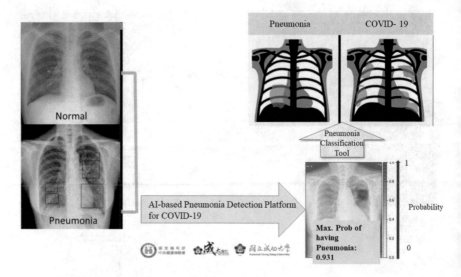

Fig. 11.7 An artificial intelligence-based pneumonia detection platform for COVID-19: MedCheX. (Source: NHI Data Warehouse Professor Jung-Hsien Chiang of National Cheng Kung University)

models were performed that lead reviewers only have to confirm those cases with inconsistency. Hereafter, the burden of professional review has been greatly alleviated, patients' medical rights have been protected, and the waiting time for drug approval has been shortened as well.

2. Development of the MedCheX

The NHIA and National Cheng Kung University Hospital jointly developed the MedCheX (Fig. 11.7). After patients' chest X-rays are taken, the doctors could upload the image to the system and then automatically obtain evaluation generated by AI models to determine the patients' risk of COVID-19 and images marked with the location of the lesion within 1 min. The system is a great example of how AI technology is utilized to assist doctors with precise diagnosis and find confirmed COVID-19 cases earlier, leading to a decrease in the risk of community spread.

Future Perspectives

The NHIA will continue to integrate structured and unstructured data into the NHI database to optimize AI tools, to develop and seek external resources to increase the effectiveness of AI tools, and to promote more diversified AI applications in the review process. Simultaneously, the NHIA is committed to gradually introducing useful AI tools in each step of the review process, with an effort to construct a comprehensively AI-assisted precision claim review system.

Chapter 12
Digital Transformation of Big Data

Po-Chang Lee, Chih-Hsing Ho, and Joyce Tsung-Hsi Wang

Introduction

The National Health Insurance (NHI), the single-payer system, not only protects the right to access to health care for Taiwan's residents, but also centralizes and coordinates resources and regulates their wide range of applications. The system has won international praise for its advantages of low administrative costs, fairness and consistency of insurance premiums and has become a reference model for other countries when establishing or reforming their health insurance systems. In recent times, the NHI has been undergoing a digital transformation by combining digital technology and the concepts of data governance. It is hoped that the NHI will provide high-quality medical care for the public under the premise of limited resources and continuously move toward the ultimate goal of Universal Health Coverage (UHC) proposed by the World Health Organization (WHO).

Issues: People's Consent to Data Authorization Collection [1]

In 2012, the Taiwan Association for Human Rights filed a lawsuit against the Health Insurance Administration (NHIA), arguing that the medical records of the NHI cannot be provided to researchers and academic organizations without people's consent and explicit authorization by law. Although the NHIA won the lawsuit because of public interests, this argument is under review by the Constitutional Court.

P.-C. Lee (✉) · J. T.-H. Wang
National Health Insurance Administration, Ministry of Health and Welfare, Taipei, Taiwan
e-mail: pochang@nhi.gov.tw; mdjoyce@nhi.gov.tw

C.-H. Ho
Institute of European and American Studies, Academia Sinica, Taipei, Taiwan
e-mail: chihho@gate.sinica.edu.tw

© The Author(s) 2022
P.-C. Lee et al. (eds.), *Digital Health Care in Taiwan*,
https://doi.org/10.1007/978-3-031-05160-9_12

The NHIA has a huge database, with a collection of more than 70 billion records of medical data accumulated over the past 27 years. Since 2018, by collecting medical images, including computed tomography (CT) and magnetic resonance imaging (MRI), and the analysis and value-added applications of the NHI big data, the NHI database has become the cornerstone for developing the precision medicine and biotechnology industry.

The NHIA has great concerns about the legitimacy of the secondary use of the NHI data and personal information protection. It is essential that the release of the NHI data is legitimate and that these de-identified data are pseudonymized or anonymized.

People tend to regard pseudonymized data as anonymized data. However, according to the US Health Insurance Portability and Accountability Act, 18 items of personal identification fields (identifier) must be removed to achieve de-identification. Thus, the NHIA still has a long way to go.

The EU General Data Protection Regulation (GDPR) states that pseudonymized personal data still constitute one kind of personal data. In Taiwan, medical data and insurance data were uploaded to the NHI system, and personal identification fields were encrypted. Although completely removing personal data may avoid data being identified, there is still a possibility of data leakage. If too many personal data are deleted, it may not be easy to use academic research and value-added applications.

According to the Personal Data Protection Act (PDPA), personal data, including medical records, medical services, genetics, and health examinations, shall not be collected, processed, or used. However, this Act also points out that government agencies and academic institutions are not limited to health care, public health, and crime prevention. It should be guaranteed that the specific individuals cannot be identified by data processing.

The NHIA has developed the My Health Bank system for people and the National Health Insurance MediCloud System (NHI MediCloud System) for physicians and pharmacists to facilitate data use. More than seven million people have used the My Health Bank system to check up on personal medical records.

The NHIA has repeatedly stated that the rationale of the secondary use of the NHI data is based on the public interests and the use must be in accordance with the law. In fact, it is essential for people to be fully informed and then the NHIA must obtain their consent. Therefore, one questionnaire in the National Health Insurance Mobile Easy Access mobile application (NHI Express app) is provided for users to express their willingness to consent to the use of their own personal medical records.

Taiwan's NHI adopts a single-payer system. The claims data collected over the past 27 years are among the country's precious assets. Facing the issues of human rights protection, the point of balance must be reached between innovations and securing people's rights. Further, making good and proper use of the NHI data cannot be avoided in the face of public interests.

National Health Insurance Open Data and Personal Data Protection—Challenges and Prospects of the Secondary Use of Health Data [2]

Chih-Hsing Ho

In 2020, the NHIA revised its rules on the NHI Database Application Service to include commercial access to de-identified data of 3.5 million deceased individuals. This plan to unlock data has sparked controversy. The NHIA has consequently suspended this policy implementation to wait for social consensus.

It has been argued that deceased individuals are not natural persons to be protected by the data protection law and that the public benefits of open data should be recognized. However, it remains arguable whether there are sufficient legal grounds for the secondary use of the deceased's health data beyond its primary purpose. In Taiwan, the original purpose of collecting NHI data is for premium auditing only. As the deceased individuals had not had a chance to consent to data reuse while they were alive, opening up their health data for secondary purposes requires a lawful basis.

According to Paragraph 4, as a proviso of Article 6 of the PDPA in Taiwan, "public service agencies" or "academic research institutions" may use de-identified data for health or medical purposes. This rule sets restrictions on a limited set of applicant entities so that commercial entities need to rely on a public–private collaboration to apply for access to NHI data.

Even though the NHIA had once revised its internal rules to expand data access to commercial entities, such administrative rules are not up to the legislation level. In addition, even if there is a requirement for approval from institutional review boards (IRBs) for data access, it remains arguable whether it is appropriate to rely on the amendment of the administrative rules to bypass the PDPA. Overall, relying on internal rules would not be a long-term solution to the NHI Open Database.

Furthermore, the EU GDPR stipulates that pseudonymized data remain personal data to be protected. According to the GDPR, the process of de-identification is regarded as an appropriate safeguard for data processing that cannot "replace consent" as a sufficient condition or a lawful basis for the reuse of data. In practice, the operating standard for evaluating how the data have been processed to be "non-identifiable" remains to be established in Taiwan. If the data are not truly "anonymous," according to the EU standards, they are still personal data and fall within the scope of the GDPR.

Thus, are there any possible ways to expand access to the secondary use of the NHI data? The advice can be mapped out in the following five directions:

1. Incorporate a dynamic consent model in the My Health Bank app to allow individuals to consent to the secondary use of their health data. It includes marking their preferences for different types of data, sharing scenarios, applying entities,

and access purposes that shall be managed through the sophisticated IT system and modified at any time.

2. Stipulate special laws or allow individuals to opt out of their data being used for research or commercial purposes if made accessible. For example, the Health and Social Care Act 2012 is the legal basis for National Health Service (NHS) Digital's legal right to collect health data in England. This bill is supplemented by a National Data Opt-Out Programme that allows patients to opt out of their confidential information to be used for research and planning.

3. Refer to the EU GDPR to amend the PDPA in Taiwan. It is advised to set restrictions on "data usage purposes" rather than "applicant entities" to allow private entities to access de-identified data so long as the data processing and use is for the public interest, or for scientific or statistical purposes.

4. Set up a data access committee for data access control and management. It is advised to classify risks associated with different data types and carry out privacy impact assessment and independent ethical review prior to granting access to data.

5. Refer to benefit-sharing arrangements adopted by the NHS on its public-private partnerships. It is advised to require a certain percentage of commercial benefits to be returned to the NHI Fund to balance private interests and public benefits. The purpose is to gain more social trust when considering expanding access to NHI data for commercial use.

Prospects of the Use of NHI Data

The NHI database has so far accumulated more than 70 billion medical records and 3.4 billion medical images. This immense medical database is a precious national asset. The NHI has improved people's health and wellbeing; its valuable database will help precision medicine and digital health and related industries to thrive. However, although confronted with the conflicts among innovative values, the interests of using medical big data, and human rights issues, the NHIA will find a balance between pioneering and conservative policies more pragmatically and create an environment that is more conducive to the health and happiness of the next generation.

In order to have an open communication with the public, the NHIA has started a "use and sharing the NHI data" survey in "My Health Bank," which has nearly seven million users, to collect public opinions on using the NHI data for academic, research, and commercial purposes. From 9 July 2021 to 18 October 2021, more than 80,000 people filled out the survey. Among them, 92% support the use of encrypted NHI data for academic and research purposes, and 85% support expanding the data access to commercial entities, hoping to facilitate the development of digital technology.

In order to be in line with the EU GDRP, the NHIA has conducted the "Personal Data Use Notification Consent" trial survey. More than 50,000 people expressed their willingness to make decisions on their personal NHI data. If options are given in the future, more than 82% of the people are willing to provide their personal health data for academic use; 83% of the respondents agree that the NHIA should open access to personal data for commercial entities under the condition that personal data are completely de-identified and it should be impossible to identify individuals.

The preliminary survey found that 80% of the respondents have a positive attitude toward the application of the NHI data, which shows that people have confidence in the importance of the NHI data for industry development. The NHIA will continue the public communication for the policy of opening up the NHI data to strengthen social trust. We look forward to driving the digital transformation of Taiwan's healthcare industry through public-private partnership and cross-domain cooperation to enhance the health and well-being of the people.

Academic Applications of the National Health Insurance Database

The medical claims data have been stored in the medical data warehouse built by the NHIA since 1995. The data accumulated over 27 years include the medical information of all insured people in Taiwan. Unlike Medicare and Medicaid in the United States, which only include subsets of the population, or the NHS in the United Kingdom, in which people can opt-out of the centralized database, the NHI's data system is a medical database of the whole population, representing the real-world data of people receiving medical services in Taiwan. To promote the development of medical and health care, the NHIA offers encrypted and de-identified NHI data to academic institutions and healthcare researchers to apply, while protecting people's privacy rights, data security, and reasonable use. Many academic research results have been published in academic journals. Furthermore, to promote the sharing of NHI data and reduce the duplication of resources invested, the NHIA has compiled 6550 international journal articles published from 2005 to 2021 that utilized Taiwan's NHI data and has established a search engine for these articles. They are classified into ten categories, including "biochemistry, genetics, and molecular biology," "dentistry," "health professions, immunology, and microbiology," "medicine," "neuroscience," "nursing," "pharmacology," "toxicology and pharmaceutics," "psychology," and "social sciences. " The search engine is designed in a user-friendly and intuitive way. Users can directly apply filters for keywords, journal, article title, author, publication period or subject and easily search for journal articles using Taiwan's NHI data on the official website of the NHIA.

In addition to displaying bibliographic information, the query results also direct the users to the PubMed website for the full text so that researchers or those who are interested in using the NHI database can quickly learn from the experience of previous researchers. The previous studies are "the shoulders of giants" that we can stand on to improve the effectiveness of our studies.

Development and Planning of Decision Aid Tools

According to the WHO Digital Health Guideline released in 2019, the intervention of digital technologies, such as mobile phones, tablets, and computers, improves people's health and strengthens necessary services, which are critical components in achieving the goal of UHC. Because Taiwan's NHI database has rare and valuable evidence-based data, the NHIA launched the "NHI Big Data Digital Application Project" to introduce artificial intelligence (AI) into the system and develop decision aid tools through information and communication technology and the integration of mobility, cloud computing, and big data.

For healthcare providers, the clinical decision support system enables physicians to make more precise decisions regarding clinical treatment, providing a solid foundation for the development of precision medicine and holistic health care. For example, physicians can evaluate follow-up medication more accurately by reviewing the monitoring record of patients' personal blood international normalized ratio (INR). By tracking personal health status, patient decision aids (PDA) serve as a reference for patients or the general public when they make self-care decisions, such as blood sugar control during pregnancy and suggestions on how to deal with COVID-19-induced emotions for adolescents.

Under the core value of data governance, the NHIA combines the NHI database and emerging technologies to establish smart medical care services, hoping to address health issues that are of concern to medical providers and people and provide people with more convenient and efficient services with digital technology. In response to the core concept of smart government development, the NHIA continues to improve public services with open data and implement "open data transparency and maximized value-added applications" to achieve goals of continuous quality improvement of medical care services and more efficient use of medical resources.

Developing Virtual NHI Cards to Meet the Needs of Atypical Medical Fields

The Virtual NHI Card falls under the big project of Smart Government, which supports the development of "Digital Nation." In line with the national digital transformation and in response to the need for digital healthcare, the NHIA has virtualized the NHI cards and expanded the virtual NHI Card Pilot Project in 2021. People can now use the virtual NHI card when seeking medical treatment in atypical medical

Smart Government Supports the National Digital Transformation

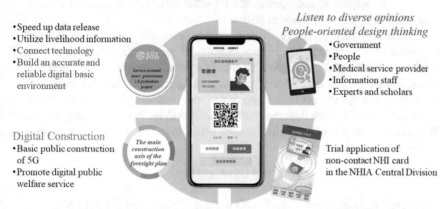

Listen to diverse opinions
People-oriented design thinking

• Speed up data release
• Utilize livelihood information
• Connect technology
• Build an accurate and reliable digital basic environment

• Government
• People
• Medical service provider
• Information staff
• Experts and scholars

Digital Construction
• Basic public construction of 5G
• Promote digital public welfare service

The main construction axis of the foresight plan

Trial application of non-contact NHI card in the NHIA Central Division

Fig. 12.1 The virtual NHI card supports the development of "Digital Nation"

fields, such as "home-based medical care," "teleconsultations," and "telecommunications." (Fig. 12.1).

By the end of 2019, the COVID-19 pandemic deeply impacted the healthcare and medical systems in many countries. The healthcare industry has introduced Information Technology to upgrade their service models and provide solutions for safer and easier ways of delivering medical care. The virtual NHI card is an excellent example of how physical contact can be reduced when combining telecommunications and medical care to improve convenience and reduce the risk for people seeking medical care.

The use of the virtual NHI card through the entire outpatient visit flow, including registration, consultation, and medicine pick-up, has been fully tested. The NHIA will continue to refine the service process to improve connectivity and comprehension. Multiple virtual NHI card reading methods will be developed, such as self-scanning and scanning by mobile device camera, to decrease the necessity of a QR code scanner, hoping to establish a more convenient and safer service model.

To optimize the convenience of home-based medical care, the NHIA added the virtual NHI card QR code function to the "home-based medical care Bluetooth App" in August 2021. Before leaving their facilities to provide home-based medical care services, medical professionals can complete the authentication of the medical institution card and medical staff card first. At the patient's home, they only have to scan a patient's virtual NHI card's QR code through the Bluetooth App to query the NHI MediCloud System, give a consultation, and upload the data. In this way, the equipment that medical professionals need to carry for home-based medical care will be reduced and the process will be simplified.

In the future, the NHIA will leverage the full-scale roll-out of the virtual NHI cards for "home-based medical care" to meet the medical needs of the public and medical institutions and gradually expand the implementation to cover all services that the NHI provides. In the long term, the use of the virtual NHI card will be expanded to outpatient, emergency, and inpatient settings to comprehensively promote their utilization for medical treatment.

The development of the virtual NHI card protects the right to receive medical treatment of people residing in remote areas or areas with insufficient medical resources. It also plays an important role in epidemic prevention by meeting the medical needs during the epidemic. In the post-epidemic era, the development of a digital medical system can reduce the risk of unnecessary exposure during medical treatment and reduce the burden on the medical system. We believe that the virtual NHI card will be a useful tool for identity verification and will become a powerful platform for public services.

Artificial Intelligence Application Pilot Project of National Health Insurance Data

From 2018 to 2020, the NHIA and the National Development Council jointly implemented the Asia Silicon Valley Development Plan to promote the application of AI in medical imaging. This project, which was divided into three phases, gradually opens the NHI data up to external organizations for value-added applications through an industry–academia cooperation mechanism. Therefore, the NHIA started the "NHI Data AI Application Services Pilot Project" in June 2019 to embody the core value of the plan, promoting the NHI data sharing and social innovation services while protecting personal health privacy. The plan allows academic and research units to team up with industry and apply for de-identified medical images, such as CT and MRI, to test or develop AI application models.

The purpose, rationality, and relevance of each team's proposal must be viewed by the NHI Data AI Application Review Committee, and the de-identification mechanism must be confirmed to guarantee that no individual can be recognized before the team can access the NHI image data in the designated locations. A total of 15 teams participated, including 9 medical organizations and 6 academic institutions, and 10 were collaborations between industry and academia.

The research designs of the teams mainly included AI model verification and construction. The former is for research teams to verify the validity of the AI model developed with single data sources with real-world data or adjust the model parameters through the NHI database to broaden the model's applicability. The latter uses the NHI big data to develop AI models. The main research topics include a disease prediction reference model, auxiliary verification, and correction of medical image location and lesion interpretation, establishment of an early disease prediction model, enhancement of computer image organ segmentation and labelling model validation, postoperative risk prediction model data expansion, as well as prediction of the incidence of lifestyle-related diseases.

The AI models developed or verified by the participating teams have achieved outstanding results. Among them, the world's first AI pancreas diagnosis auxiliary tool, PANCREASaver, which provides early warnings of pancreatic cancer, was published in a top international journal—*The Lancet Digital Health*. One medical institution has introduced AI models and coordinated them with the green channel mechanism to arrange inspections in hospitals. With the assistance of AI, the patient's brain metastases can be accurately identified early. Moreover, by largely reducing the patient's waiting time from initial diagnosis examination to return visits for reports, doctors can utilize the golden treatment period and achieve better outcomes. Another successful example is the "Chest X-Ray Image Assisted Research System for COVID-19," which the NHIA and National Cheng Kung University developed jointly. The system uses de-identified X-ray images of COVID-19 in the NHI database to balance the performance of the images from different disease stages. The system can detect COVID-19 with an accuracy rate of 92%. In the future, the NHIA will integrate an image AI service on the virtual private network platform for medical institutions to upload chest X-ray images and leverage the power of the "Image AI National Team." Such a "scientific and technological anti-epidemic sentinel" mechanism adds value to the epidemic prevention technology developed.

With the ageing of the population and the changing of lifestyles, the application of innovative technologies, such as information communication and AI, to change the delivery of medical services is one of the most crucial issues internationally. In response to expectations from the public, the NHIA opened the second phase of the "NHI Data AI Application Service Center Pilot Project" in March 2021. By mid-September 2021, three teams had submitted applications and successively participated. To provide more convenient medical services, the NHIA plans to discuss the important results with the research team and evaluate the feasibility of introducing their technology to the NHIA. This will improve the effectiveness of the NHI medical claim reviews and enable the NHIA to provide AI-assisted models on public platforms for all medical institutions to use so that the whole population can receive better medical care.

Conclusion

The importance of the NHI big data and its research contribution is non-negligible. The claims data collected in the past 27 years are among the country's precious assets. Facing the issues of human rights protection, the point of balance must be reached between innovations and securing people's rights. Further, making good and proper use of the NHI data cannot be avoided in the fact of the public interest. The NHIA will continue to find a balance to open up NHI data for research use, aiming to drive the development of related industries and promote the growth of innovative and accurate smart medical systems and health aid tools. By adding value to health data, collective statistical information can have application value.

Through resource sharing, activation, and reuse, we can maximize the value of health data. The NHI will utilize medical AI lawfully and carefully to launch a new era of smart medical care that benefits all people.

References

1. Po-Chang Lee, 20210705 健康名人堂, United Daily News.
2. Chih-Hsing Ho, 20210322 健康名人堂, United Daily News.

Appendix: National Health Insurance Act

Amended Date: 2021-01-20

Chapter 1 General Principles

Article 1

The purpose of this Act is to promote the health of all nationals, to administer the National Health Insurance (hereinafter referred to as 'this Insurance'), and to provide health services.

This Insurance is compulsory social Insurance. Benefits shall be provided during the Insured term under the provisions of this Act in the event of illness, injury, or maternity occurring to the beneficiary.

Article 2

Terms used in this Act are defined as follows:

1. Beneficiary refers to the Insured and his/her dependents.
2. Dependents refers to:

    (a) The Insured's spouse, who is not employed;
    (b) The Insured's lineal blood ascendants, who are not employed;
    (c) The Insured's lineal blood descendants, within the second degree of relationship, who are either minors and not employed, or are incapable of making a living, including those who are in school and not employed.

© National Health Insurance Administration, Ministry of Health and Welfare, Taiwan 2022
P.-C. Lee et al. (eds.), *Digital Health Care in Taiwan*,
https://doi.org/10.1007/978-3-031-05160-9

3. Premium Withholder refers to an individual from whom the premium is withheld, according to taxation law.
4. Benefit Payments refers to the remainder of total medical benefit payments, less the self-borne medical fees of the Insured, based on the Act.
5. Insurance Budget refers to the Insurance benefit expenditures and reserve funds that should be established or added.
6. Medical Visit Advice refers to the process of understanding the Insured's medical visit practices when they have duplicated medical visits, undergone repetitive visits, or used inappropriate treatment. It involves providing appropriate medical and health education, and arranging and assisting with medical visits.

Article 3

The Government should bear at least 36% of the remainder of the annual Insurance Budget, less promulgated revenues.

The Government must include in the budget 36% of the deficit remainder of the annual Insurance Budget, less promulgated revenues. The Competent Authority shall draw up a budget to cover the deficit.

Article 4

The Competent Authority of this Insurance shall be the Ministry of Health and Welfare.

Article 5

The National Health Insurance Committee (hereinafter referred to as the 'NHIC') shall be responsible for the following tasks:

1. Review of premiums;
2. Review of the scope of benefits;
3. Coordination of drafting and allocation of medical benefit payments;
4. Study and interpretation of Insurance laws and policies;
5. Other supervisory functions pertaining to Insurance matters.

If the NHIC determines a reduction in Insurance revenues or an increase in Insurance expenditure, the NHIC, as the Insurer, should present a proposal for resource allocation and financial balance, to be reviewed and coordinated jointly.

The NHIC should publish its agenda for any meeting to review and coordinate matters relevant to this Insurance. The minutes should be published within 10 days after the meeting. Before reviewing and coordinating major matters, the NHIC should gather information on public opinion and, if necessary, organise related activities involving the public.

The NHIC is composed of Insured persons, employers, Insurance medical service providers, experts, reputable public figures, and representatives from relevant agencies. Representatives from premium payers should not be less than half of the total number of NHIC members. Representatives from beneficiaries should be not less than one-third of the total number of NHIC members.

The Competent Authority shall determine the number of members, how they are selected, the regulations for meetings, self-disclosure of representatives' interest, and disclosure to the public.

Matters reviewed and coordinated by the NHIC should be approved by the Competent Authority or presented to the Executive Yuan for approval. Matters approved by the Executive Yuan should be sent to the Legislative Yuan for future reference.

Article 6

The Insured, the Group Insurance Applicant, the Premium Withholder, and the Contracted Medical Institution may apply for a review to settle a dispute against the Insurer. They may file an administrative appeal or an administrative lawsuit if they disagree with the review's findings.

The National Health Insurance Dispute Mediation Committee shall perform the task of reviewing such disputes.

The Competent Authority shall determine the scope of the abovementioned disputes, applications for review, deadlines for submission of documents, procedures, methods, and processes.

The National Health Insurance Dispute Mediation Committee shall publish dispute review results periodically, through publication in a Government gazette, on the Internet, or through other proper methods.

Publication of dispute review results shall be performed after information relating to individuals, groups, and judicial entities has been de-identified through coding, anonymising, redacting, or other methods, and is no longer identifiable.

Chapter 2 The Insurer, The Beneficiary, and The Group Insurance Applicant

Article 7

The Insurer of this Insurance shall be the National Health Insurance Administration, Ministry of Health and Welfare, which will administer the Insurance business.

Article 8

Any national of the Republic of China must meet one of the following requirements in order to become a beneficiary of this Insurance:

1. Those who have subscribed to this Insurance within the last 2 years and have a registered domicile in Taiwan, or those with an established, registered domicile in the Taiwan area for at least 6 consecutive months prior to subscription to this Insurance;
2. The following individuals with established registered domiciles in the Taiwan area at the time of becoming a subscriber:

    (a) Civil servants or full-time and regularly paid personnel in governmental agencies and public and private schools;
    (b) Employees of publicly or privately owned enterprises or institutions;
    (c) Employees, other than those prescribed in the preceding two items, of particular employers;
    (d) Newborns in the Taiwan area;
    (e) The spouses and offspring of Government officials assigned abroad.

Individuals who have previously subscribed to this Insurance and have gone abroad before this revision was promulgated (4 January 2011) should immediately establish residency and subscribe to this Insurance when they return to the country. Within 1 year of the revision being implemented, they will not be subject to the 6-month restriction specified in Subparagraph 1 above.

Article 9

With the exception of individuals specified in Article 8, any person in the Taiwan area who has an Alien Resident Certificate must meet one of the following requirements in order to become a beneficiary of this Insurance:

1. Those with an established, registered domicile in Taiwan for at least 6 months;
2. Those with a regular employer;
3. Newborns in the Taiwan area.

Article 10

The Insured shall be classified into the following six categories.

1. Category 1:

    (a) Civil servants or full-time and regularly paid personnel in Government agencies and public and private schools;
    (b) Employees of publicly or privately owned enterprises or institutions;

   (c) Employees, other than those included in the preceding two items, who are employed by particular employers;

   (d) Employers or self-employed business owners;

   (e) Independently practicing professionals and technicians.

2. Category 2:

   (a) Members of an occupational union who have no particular employer, or who are self-employed;

   (b) Seamen serving on foreign vessels, who are members of the National Seamen's Union or the Master Mariners' Association.

3. Category 3:

   (a) Members of the Farmers' Association or the Irrigation Association, or workers older than 15 years who are actively engaged in agricultural activities;

   (b) Class A members of the Fishers' Association who are either self-employed or have no particular employer, or workers older than 15 years who are engaged in fishery activities.

4. Category 4:

   (a) Military servicemen whose compulsory service terms are longer than 2 months or who are summoned to serve for longer than 2 months, military school students who receive grants from the Government, the descendants of military servicemen who lost their support from the Ministry of Defence, and the descendants of deceased servicemen who receive associated pensions;

   (b) Men of age for enlistment in the military, who are in military-substitute service;

   (c) Those who are serving sentences in correctional institutions or receiving punishments from police and military courts martial. This is not applicable to those serving sentences of less than 2 months or under parole conditions.

5. Category 5:
Household members of low-income families, as defined by the Social Support Law.

6. Category 6:

   (a) Veterans and household representatives of survivors of veterans;

   (b) Representatives or heads of households, other than the Insured or their dependents, as prescribed in Subparagraphs 1–5 and the preceding item of this Subparagraph.

The standard for identification and qualification of workers actually engaged in agricultural activities under item (1) of Subparagraph 3 and workers actually engaged in fishery activities under item (2) of Subparagraph 3 shall be established jointly by the Central Agricultural Competent Authority and the Competent Authority.

Article 11

The Insured classified in Category 1 may not opt for reclassification to Category 2 or Category 3. The Insured classified in Category 2 may not opt for reclassification to Category 3. The Insured classified in Categories 1–3 may not opt for reclassification to Categories 4–6. However, Class A members of the Fishers Association who hire 10 or fewer labourers for ocean fishing and are actually engaged in fishery activities should be classified as Category 3 from 21 January 2002.

Those who qualified as Insured shall not subscribe to this Insurance as dependents.

Article 12

The dependents of the Insured specified in Article 2 shall subscribe to or withdraw from this Insurance together with the Insured. However, this rule shall not be applicable to situations that are recognised by the Competent Authority as making it difficult for dependents to subscribe to or withdraw from this Insurance together with the Insured, including, but not limited to, situations of domestic abuse.

Article 13

The following persons are not covered by this Insurance and shall be withdrawn from it if they have subscribed to this Insurance:

1. Those who have been missing for 6 months or longer;
2. Those who are not qualified under Articles 8 or 9.

Article 14

The commencement of the Insurance shall take effect from the date of occurrence of qualification, as specified in Articles 8 and 9.

The termination of the Insurance shall take effect from the date of occurrence of the previous Article.

Article 15

The Group Insurance Applicants for the different categories of Insured are as follows:

1. For the Insured in Categories 1 and 2, their Group Insurance Applicants shall be the agencies, schools, enterprises, institutions, or employers they work for, or the unions of which they are members. The Group Insurance Applicants that cover

the Insured in the Ministry of Defence shall be designated by the Ministry of Defence.

2. For the Insured in Category 3, the Group Insurance Applicants shall be the lowest-level Farmers Association, Irrigation Association, or Fishers Association to which they belong, or located at the place where the Insured's household is registered.

3. For the Insured in Category 3, the Group Insurance Applicants are as follows:

   (a) For the Insured in item 1, Subparagraph 4, Paragraph 1, Article 10, the Group Insurance Applicants shall be designated by the Ministry of Defence.

   (b) For the Insured in item 2, Subparagraph 4, Paragraph 1, Article 10, the Group Insurance Applicants shall be designated by the Ministry of Interior.

   (c) For the Insured in item 3, Subparagraph 4, Paragraph 1, Article 10, the Group Insurance Applicants shall be designated by the Ministry of Justice and the Ministry of Defence.

   (d) For the Insured in Categories 5 and 6, the Group Insurance Applicants may be the administration offices of the village, township, municipality, or district of their registered domicile. Otherwise, the Group Insurance Applicants may be public or private social welfare service institutions.

The Insured prescribed in item 2, Subparagraph 6, Paragraph 1 of Article 10 and their dependents may, upon consent of the Group Insurance Applicants of an Insured in another category, who live together with the above Insured and their dependents, use such units as defined by their Group Insurance Applicants, provided that the premiums shall be calculated separately, according to the provision of Article 23.

The Group Insurance Applicants prescribed in Subparagraph 4, Paragraph 1 of this Article shall set up special units or agents to administer matters relevant to this Insurance.

For any person covered under Category 6 and undergoing vocational training or training in exam-taking at a Government-registered institution, such training institution or agency shall be the Group Insurance Applicant.

If the Group Insurance Applicant fails to make premium payments for more than 2 months, the Insurer may contact another Group Insurance Applicant to administer matters related to this Insurance.

The Group Insurance Applicant shall subscribe to the Insurer for coverage within 3 days from the date on which the beneficiary met the conditions of this Insurance, and shall withdraw from the coverage within 3 days from the date of occurrence of the cause of withdrawal.

Article 16

The Insurer must produce and distribute a National Health Insurance card that has an electronic information processing function to allow it to store and send information relating to the Insured. The card may not store information that is not used for medical care purposes or information that is unrelated to the Insured receiving Insurance and medical services.

The Insurer shall charge a fee for changing or replacing the abovementioned card. It shall determine the production, issue, and replacement of the card, as well as the type, exchange, and use of information it stores and sends. The Insurer shall manage the card's use, as well as other relevant matters, which shall be announced after approval by the Competent Authority.

Chapter 3 Insurance Finance

Article 17

The Central Government, the Group Insurance Applicant, and the Insured shall jointly bear the cost of the Insurance Budget, after promulgated revenues have been deducted.

Article 18

The premium payable by the Insured and their dependents in Categories 1–3 shall be calculated according to the Insured's payroll-related amount and their premium rate. The premium rate shall be set at a maximum of 6%.

The premium payable by the Insured's dependents shall be paid by the Insured. When there are more than three dependents, the premium shall be calculated on the basis of three dependents.

Article 19

For those Insured in Categories 1–3, the Insured's payroll-related amount shall be subject to a Grading Table, drafted by the Competent Authority. The Grading Table must be submitted to the Executive Yuan for approval.

The Insured's minimum payroll-related amount in the Grading Table shall be equal to the base salary promulgated by the Central Competent Authority in charge of labour affairs. Upon adjustment of the base salary, such a minimum shall be adjusted accordingly.

The payroll-related amount at the top level of the Grading Table must be maintained at five times greater than the amount at the bottom level. The Grading Table must be revised within 1 month after the base salary is adjusted. Upon the number of Insured persons at the highest level of the Grading Table exceeding 3% of the total number of Insured persons for 12 consecutive months, the Competent Authority shall adjust the Grading Table, beginning the following month.

Article 20

The Insured payroll-related amount for the Insured in Categories 1 and 2 is determined based on the following:

1. Employees: the payroll;
2. Employers and self-employed: the business income;
3. Self-employed individuals and independently practicing professionals and technicians: the income from professional practice.

If the Insured prescribed in Categories 1 and 2 has no stable income, the Insured shall select the proper Insured payroll-related amount from the Grading Table. Such Insured payroll-related amount shall be examined by the Insurer, who may adjust it at their own discretion if the Insured payroll-related amount is found to be inappropriate.

Article 21

For the Insured under Categories 1 and 2 of the previous Article, if the income is adjusted between February and July of the current year, the Group Insurance Applicants shall notify the Insurer of the adjusted Insured payroll-related amount by the end of August of the same year. If the adjustment is made between August of the current year and January of the following year, the Group Insurance Applicants shall notify the Insurer of the adjusted Insured payroll-related amount by the end of February of the following year. This shall become effective on the first day of the month following notification.

Unless the Insured payroll-related amount, as prescribed in the preceding paragraph, has reached the highest level of this Insurance, such amount shall not be lower than the monthly labour pension reserve deposit or the Insured salary of any other social Insurance schemes to which the Insured has subscribed. If the Insured payroll-related amount of this Insurance is less than these benefits, the Group Insurance Applicant shall advise the Insurer to make the appropriate adjustment. The Insurer may make adjustment at its own discretion.

Article 22

The Insured payroll-related amount applicable to the Insured in Category 3 shall be the average amount for those specified under items 2 and 3 of Subparagraph 1, and Subparagraph 2 of Paragraph 1, Article 10. The Insurer may adjust the level of the Insured payroll-related amount according to the financial position of the Insured and their dependents.

Article 23

The premiums of those Insured in Categories 4–6 shall be calculated according to the averaged actuarial premium, based on the total number of beneficiaries, in accordance with Article 18.

The premiums of such dependents shall be paid by the Insured. When there are more than three dependents, the payment shall be calculated on the basis of three dependents.

Article 24

The Insurer should apply for a review at a meeting of the NHIC 1 month after the premium rate of beneficiaries and dependents in Article 18 are determined. If premiums at the maximum rate do not balance with the medical benefit payments approved for the year, negotiations regarding the total amount of medical benefit payments should be conducted.

Before its annual review, the NHIC should invite actuaries, Insurance and finance experts, economists, and reputable public figures to provide opinions.

In accordance with the negotiations, the NHIC's review should draft the total amount of medical benefit payments 1 month before the start of the year, completing the review of balance of payment rates. This shall be reported to the Competent Authority, which will, in turn, report it to the Executive Yuan for approval before announcing it publicly. If the review cannot be completed within the specified time, the Competent Authority shall report this matter to the Executive Yuan for approval before announcing it publicly.

Article 25

The Insurer shall perform an actuarial process for premium finance at least once every 5 years, with each such actuarial process covering a period of 25 years.

Article 26

Upon the occurrence of any of the following events in this Insurance, the Insurer shall adjust the premium rate and present it to the NHIC, which shall report it to the Competent Authority and then to the Executive Yuan for approval, after which, the Competent Authority shall announce it publicly:

1. The reserve fund of this Insurance falls below the total Insurance benefit amount for 1 month.
2. There is any addition to, or reduction in, benefit items, contents, or payment schedules that affects the financial balance of this Insurance.

Chapter 4 Collection and Calculation of Premiums

Article 27

The contribution rates for this Insurance shall be calculated according to the following provisions of Articles 18 and 23:

1. For the Insured in Category 1:

    (a) The Insured and their dependents referred to in item 1, Subparagraph 1, Paragraph 1 of Article 10 shall pay 30% of the premium, with the other 70% of it paid by the Group Insurance Applicants. For Insured who are employees of private schools, they and their dependents shall pay 30%, with 35% being paid by their employers and the remaining 35% being subsidised by the Central Government.

    (b) The Insured and their dependents referred to in items 2 and 3 of Subparagraph 1, Paragraph 1 of Article 10 shall pay 30% of the premium, the Group Insurance Applicants paying 60% and the remaining 10% being subsidised by the Central Government.

    (c) The Insured and their dependents referred to in items 4 and 5 of Subparagraph 1, Paragraph 1 of Article 10 shall pay the full premium.

2. The Insured and their dependents in Category 2 shall pay 60% of the premium, with the remaining 40% being subsidised by the Central Government.

3. The Insured and their dependents in Category 3 shall pay 30% of the premium, with the remaining 70% being subsidised by the Central Government.

4. For the Insured in Category 4:

    (a) For the Insured in item 1, Subparagraph 4, Paragraph 1 of Article 10, their institutions shall subsidise their premiums in full.

    (b) For the Insured in item 2, Subparagraph 4, Paragraph 1, Article 10, the Central Military Training Administrative Authority shall subsidise the premium in full.

    (c) For the Insured in item 3, Subparagraph 4, Paragraph 1 of Article 10, the Central Correctional Authority and the Ministry of Defence shall subsidise the premium in full.

5. For the Insured in Category 5, the Central Competent Authority in charge of social welfare shall subsidise the premium in full.

6. The premium payable by the Insured referred to in item 1, Subparagraph 6, Paragraph 1 of Article 10 shall be subsidised by the Veterans Affairs Commission of the Executive Yuan; 30% of the premium of the Insured and their dependents shall be self-covered, with 70% subsidised by the Veterans Affairs Commission.

7. The Insured and their dependents referred to in item 2, Subparagraph 6, Paragraph 1 of Article 10 shall pay 60% of the premium, with the Central Government subsidising 40%.

Article 28

Before the promulgation of this amendment on 4 January 2011, any Government agency that has not been able to secure funds to pay the Insurer in accordance with Article 29 (pre-amendment) should present a pay-back plan to the Insurer. The time-frame for paying back should not exceed 8 years. The Insurer may request interest payments, in accordance with Article 30 (pre-amendment).

Article 29

The number of dependents in items 1–3 of Category 1, for whom the premium is subsidised by Group Insurance Applicants or the Government, shall be the average number of dependents of Insured persons in items 1–3 of Category 1.

Article 30

The premium of this Insurance shall be paid monthly, according to the provisions of Articles 18 and 23:

1. The premium to be contributed by the Insured in Category 1 shall be deducted from the payroll and paid to the Insurer by the Group Insurance Applicant, together with the Group Insurance Applicant's contributions, by the end of the following month.
2. The premium to be contributed by the Insured in Categories 2, 3, and 6 shall be paid monthly to their Group Insurance Applicant. The Group Insurance Applicant shall forward the accumulated premiums to the Insurer no later than the end of the following month.
3. The premium payable by the Insured in Category 5 shall be paid by the Central Competent Authority to the Insurer no later than the fifth day of the current month.
4. For the Insured in Categories 1–4 and 6, the premiums shall be part-subsidised by various levels of Government, and shall be paid in advance to the Insurer twice-yearly, by the ends of January and July. The account shall be settled at the end of the year.

The premium of this Insurance shall be fully paid for the month when the Insured subscribed to coverage. It shall be exempted for the month when the Insured withdraws from coverage.

Article 31

The Insured in Categories 1–4 and 6 shall pay supplementary Insurance premiums, based on the supplementary Insurance rate, that shall be deducted by the Premium Withholder upon payment and paid to the Insurer before the end of the month following payment. However, single benefit payments in excess of 10 million New Taiwanese Dollars, and those not reaching a certain amount, are exempted from deductions.

1. Accumulated annual bonus given by Group Insurance Applicant in excess of four times the monthly premium rateable wages.
2. Salary earnings other than those from the Group Insurance Applicant. This is not applicable to the salary earnings of Category 2 Insured persons.
3. Income from professional practice. However, income from professional practice that is designated by Article 20 as Insured payroll-related amount is not to be included in the calculation of premium rateable wages.
4. Stock earnings. However, this is not applicable to premiums already included in the premium rateable wages.
5. Interest earnings.
6. Earnings from rentals.

If the deduction cannot be made within a specified time, the Premium Withholder shall pay first.

The Competent Authority shall determine the amount referred to in Paragraph 1, the method of deduction and payment of the supplementary premium, and other relevant matters.

Article 32

Those who are not eligible, who have lost their eligibility, or who are deemed as not requiring the Premium Withholder to deduct supplementary premium should notify the Premium Withholder prior to receiving benefit payments, so that no supplementary premium will be deducted.

Article 33

The supplementary premium rates of Article 31 shall be calculated, at 2%, 1 year after the implementation of the amendment of the Act on 4 January 2011. In the second year, supplementary premium rates should be adjusted in accordance with the Insurance premium rate, which shall be announced by the Competent Authority.

Article 34

For Group Insurance Applicants of items 1–3 of Category 1, when the total amount of salary paid exceeds the Insured payroll-related amount for that month, the supplementary premium should be calculated based on the difference, as well as the rate in the previous Article, and paid jointly each month in accordance with the payment structure specified in Article 27.

Article 35

A grace period of 15 days shall be permitted in cases were the Group Insurance Applicant, the Insured, or the Premium Withholder do not pay the premium during the period provided in this Act. If payment is not made by the end of the grace period, an overdue charge of 0.1% of the amount payable shall be levied, for each day of delay after the expiry date of the grace period, until the premium is fully paid, with the maximum amounts as follows:

1. 15% of the payment to be made by the Group Insurance Applicant and Premium Withholder.
2. 5% percent of the payment to be made by the Insured.

The overdue charge mentioned in the previous paragraph may be waived if it is less than the amount fixed by the Competent Authority.

If premiums and overdue charges payable by the Group Insurance Applicant/Premium Withholder remain unpaid for 30 days, the Insurer may refer the case to the Court for compulsory execution under the law; the same shall apply to an Insured who has failed to pay either the premium or the overdue charge for 150 days.

Article 36

Those who are unable to pay the premium, overdue charge, or full self-covered premium because of economic difficulties should apply to the Insurer for instalment, or apply for loans or subsidies in accordance with Article 99. The Insurer should provide assistance and, if necessary, work with social agencies or relevant professional groups to obtain assistance from within society.

The Insurer shall determine the conditions of applications, review procedures, instalment payment schedules, and other relevant matters, and report to the Competent Authority for approval and public announcement.

Article 37

The Insurer may temporarily suspend benefits for those Group Insurance Applicants or those Insured who are proven, through investigation and supervision, to have the ability to pay the premium and overdue charge but have chosen not to do so. Such restrictions do not apply to the portion of the premium payable that is withheld by or paid to the Group Insurance Applicants, those approved by the Insurer as having to be paid in instalments (according to the previous Article), or when the premium is payable during the time the Insured is receiving protection under the Domestic Violence Prevention Act.

During the temporary suspension of benefits, the premium should still be collected.

Article 38

Whenever the Group Insurance Applicants or Premium Withholder owe premium or overdue charges but have no property for execution, or do not have property to pay off their debts, the business owner(s) should be responsible for clearing the debts.

Article 39

Premiums and overdue charges of this Insurance take precedence over general claims.

Chapter 5 Insurance Benefits

Article 40

If a beneficiary encounters illness, injury, or maternity, the contracted medical care institutions shall provide medical services, drafting fee schedules, drug dispensing items, and regulations governing fee schedules pursuant to Paragraph 2 of the Medical Benefit Regulations, as well as Paragraphs 1 and 2 of Article 41.

The Competent Authority shall determine the procedures for medical visits, medical advice, provision of Insured medical services, and other regulations concerning medical services to be provided. If the Insured is in a correctional facility, the restrictions on treatment schedule and venue, as well as matters relating to guarding, transferring, and the method of providing Insurance medical services shall be determined jointly by the Competent Authority and the Ministry of Justice.

Article 41

The Fee Schedule and Reference List for Medical Services shall be established jointly by the Insurer and the relevant agencies, experts, beneficiaries, employers, and contracted medical care institutions. It shall be reported to the Competent Authority for approval.

Drug dispensing and fee schedules should be established jointly by the Insurer, relevant agencies, experts, beneficiaries, employers, and contracted medical care institutions and reported to the Competent Authority for approval. Drug providers, relevant experts, and patients should be invited to voice their opinions.

The drafting of the drug dispensing and fee schedule standards should be in accordance with the medical needs of the Insured as well as the quality of medical care. The meeting should be accurately recorded. Self-disclosure of the representatives' interests and other relevant information should be made public. The results of the Insurer's medical evaluation should be made public before the drafting process begins.

The joint drafting of the procedures in Paragraphs 1 and 2, as well as formulating the list of representatives, its selection process, term of office, disclosure of interests, and other relevant information should be determined by the Competent Authority.

Article 42

The fee schedule and reference list of medical services described in the preceding paragraph shall follow the principle of 'equal payment for same nature of illness'; the relative points shall reflect the cost of each medical service. It should be drafted taking into account volume, cases, quality, individuals, and number of days.

The Insurer may first conduct an evaluation before drafting the medical service items and fee schedule, considering human health, medical ethics, cost-effectiveness of treatment, and the finances of this Insurance. The same applies for the drafting of the drug-dispensing items and fee schedule.Some medical services and drugs are expensive, and some pose a potential danger with inappropriate use. The drug-dispensing items must be presented to the Insurer for review and approval before use, except in emergency situations.

The review items investigated before use, and the definition and reviews of emergency situations, standards, and other relevant fee schedules, should be drafted in the medical service items and fee schedule and in the drug-dispensing items and fee schedule.

Article 43

The beneficiary shall pay 20% of the expenses of either ambulatory or emergency care and 5% of home nursing care expenses. They shall pay 30%, 40%, and 50% of the expenses for direct visits without referral to outpatient departments of district hospitals, regional hospitals, and medical centres respectively.

The Insured in areas with inadequate medical resources will be exempted from paying self-borne expenses.The Competent Authority may, when necessary, sanction the collection of a fixed amount of expenses, which the beneficiaries mentioned in Paragraph 1 shall pay for, and promulgate such amount every year; such amount is to be determined in accordance with the average ambulatory care expense of the preceding year and the ratio prescribed in Paragraph 1.

The implementation of referral procedures and regulations (Paragraph 1), and the prescription of areas with inadequate medical resources (Paragraph 2), shall be regulated by the Competent Authority.

Article 44

To promote preventive medicine, implement a referral system, and improve the quality of medicine and treatment, the Insurer should draft a Family Physicians System.

The benefits of the Family Physicians System should be paid out on a per-person basis; the payment of annual benefits should be based on a patient's age, gender, illness, and other individual expenses, after correction.

The Competent Authority shall determine the implementation, regulations, and schedule of the Family Physicians System.

Article 45

The Insurer shall fix a maximum amount for special materials and a maximum amount to be paid to contracted medical care institutions. The Insurer should pay the same amount for special materials of the same functional type.

The Insured may choose a special material designated by the Insurer as being of maximum benefit, when deemed necessary by the doctor from the contracted medical care institution, and pay the difference themselves. In that case, the permit holder should apply to the Insurer, and, upon agreement with the Insurer, present jointly to the NHIC, with an implementation date, for discussion prior to submission to the Competent Authority for approval.

Article 46

The Insurer should adjust drug prices based on prevailing market conditions; prices for drugs with patents that have expired for 1 year should be reduced. Gradual adjustment to reasonable prices should be achieved within 5 years, based on prevailing market conditions.

The Competent Authority shall determine the operating procedure for the adjustment specified in the preceding paragraph, as well as the relevant rules.

Article 47

The ratio of hospitalisation expenses to be borne by beneficiaries is as follows:

1. For acute care wards: 10% for the first 30 days; 20% from the 31st to the 60th day; and 30% from the 61st day onward;
2. For chronic care wards: 5% for the first 30 days; 10% from the 31st to the 90th day; 20% from the 91st to the 180th; and 30% from the 181st day onward.

The maximum amount to be borne by the Insured for hospitalisation in an acute care ward for not more than 30 days, or in a chronic ward for not more than 180 days, for the same illness, and the maximum amount for the accumulated self-borne expenses shall be determined by the Competent Authority.

Article 48

In case of the following circumstances, the beneficiaries shall be exempted from payment of the expenses prescribed in Articles 43 and 47:

1. Major illness or injury;
2. Child delivery;
3. Receiving medical care in mountainous regions or outlying islands.

The rules relating to the exemption from the payment of expenses, as well as the major illnesses and injuries referred to in the preceding paragraph, the procedure for applying for proof of major illness and injury, and other relevant regulations shall be determined by the Competent Authority.

Article 49

The Central Competent Authority in charge of social affairs, according to Articles 43 and 47, shall prepare a budget to pay for medical visits by members of low-income households eligible under the Public Assistance Act. However, those who do not abide by referral provisions may not receive subsidies, except in special circumstances.

Article 50

Beneficiaries shall pay to the contracted medical care institutions the self-borne expenses prescribed in Articles 43 and 47.

In cases where beneficiaries fail to pay the expenses after being notified and demanded to by the contracted medical care institution, the Insurer should be notified; the Insurer may suspend benefits to the beneficiaries when necessary and, when it has been determined, through investigation and supervision that the Insured is capable but unwilling to pay. However, this is not applicable to individuals who receive protection in accordance with the Domestic Violence Prevention Act.

Article 51

Expenses arising from the following service items are not covered in this Insurance:

1. Medical service items for which the expenses shall be borne by the Government, according to other laws or regulations;
2. Immunisation and other medical services, for which the expenses shall be borne by the Government;
3. Treatment of drug addiction, cosmetic surgery, non-post-traumatic orthodontic treatment, preventive surgery, artificial reproduction, and sex conversion surgery;
4. Over-the-counter drugs and non-prescription drugs that should be used under the guidance of a physician or pharmacist;
5. Services provided by specially designated doctors, specially registered nurses, and senior registered nurses;
6. Blood, except for blood transfusion necessary for emergent injury or illness, according to the diagnosis of a doctor;
7. Human-subject clinical trials;
8. Hospital day care, except for psychiatric care;
9. Food, other than related to tube feeding and balance billing for wards;
10. Transportation, registration fees, and certificates for patients;
11. Dentures, artificial eyes, spectacles, hearing aids, wheelchairs, canes, and other treatment equipment not required for therapy;
12. Other treatments and drugs, as stipulated by the Insurer, reviewed by the NHIC, and promulgated by the Competent Authority.

Article 52

This Insurance shall not apply to a contingency incurred by war, riot, major plague or Act of God, such as severe earthquake, storm, flood, and fire, that has been identified by the Executive Yuan and provided for at all levels of Government.

Article 53

No Insurance benefits shall be paid by the Insurer for any one of the following events:

1. Excessive hospitalisation, after the Insured's refusal to be discharged from the hospital;
2. Expenses incurred from inappropriate repetitive medical visits or other improper uses of medical resources, or undergoing treatment at medical care institutions not designated by the Insurer. This restriction does not apply to medical emergencies;
3. Treatments and drugs that are not medically necessary, according to the pre-examination;
4. Violating relevant medical procedures of this Insurance.

Article 54

If the medical services provided by the contracted medical care institution to the beneficiary are determined by the Insurer to be incompatible with the provisions of this Act, the expenses may not be charged to the Insured.

Article 55

The following may apply for reimbursement by the Insurer of self-advanced medical expenses:

1. Those within the Taiwan area who visit non-contracted medical institutions because of emergency or childbirth;
2. Those outside of the Taiwan area who have a specific illness, as determined by the Insurer, and require local medical care owing to unforeseen illnesses or an emergency childbirth. The amount reimbursed should not be higher than the maximum amount set by the Competent Authority;
3. Those who received medical care services at contracted medical care institutions while their coverage was temporarily suspended but have since paid their premium in full. Those who made visits to non-contracted medical care institutions are covered by the preceding two subparagraphs;
4. Those who received treatment or gave birth in Contracted Medical Institutions and had to self-advance medical expenses, as they were not attributable to the Insured;
5. Those who covered their own expenses according to Article 47, the annual accumulation of which exceeds the maximum amount set by the Competent Authority.

Article 56

The Insured should apply for reimbursement of self-advanced medical expenses, as described in the preceding Article, according to the following deadlines:

1. Insured persons under Subparagraphs 1, 2, or 4 must apply for reimbursement of medical expenses within 6 months from the day of emergency treatment, outpatient treatment, or discharge from hospital. After the deadline, no application will be accepted. Sailors on an ocean-going fishing ship shall apply for reimbursement within 6 months from the date they return from sea.
2. Insured persons under Subparagraph 3 should apply for reimbursement within 6 months from the day relevant expenses were paid in full; this is applicable for cases within the last 5 years.
3. Insured persons under Subparagraph 5 should apply for reimbursement before 30 June of the following year.

The Competent Authority shall determine the documents required of Insured persons who apply for reimbursement of self-advanced medical expenses, the reimbursement standards and procedures, and other relevant matters.

Article 57

Under this Insurance, the Insured may not make repetitive applications for the same incident or receive duplicate payments in cash and benefits.

Article 58

From the date of withdrawal, no benefits shall be payable to beneficiaries who withdraw from coverage according to Article 13. The Insurer should return all extra premiums paid. If benefits have already been paid, the beneficiaries shall return them to the Insurer.

Article 59

The right of the beneficiary to receive cash reimbursement for self-advanced medical expenses shall not be transferred, offset, seized, or used as a security interest.

Chapter 6 Payment of Medical Expense

Article 60

The total amount of medical payments to be made under this Insurance each year shall be proposed by the Competent Authority no later than 6 months prior to the commencement of the fiscal year. After consultation with the NHIC, it shall be reported to the Executive Yuan for approval.

Article 61

No later than 3 months prior to the commencement of each fiscal year, the NHIC shall negotiate and reach the agreement on the aggregate amount of medical payments and the method of allocation, within the range of the total amount of medical payment approved by the Executive Yuan under the previous Article, and report it to the Competent Authority for approval. In cases where the NHIC does not reach an agreement in time, the Competent Authority shall make a decision at its own discretion.

The allotment for ambulatory care and hospitalisation expenses from the aggregate payment budget described in the preceding paragraph may be specified by the district.

An allocation ratio and system of separating accounts for medical and pharmaceutical expenses may be established in regard to the budget for payment of the ambulatory care described in the preceding paragraph, according to the ambulatory care services provided by physicians, Chinese medicine doctors and dentists, pharmaceutical services, and for the expense of drugs.

After the benefit expense package in Paragraph 1 has been drafted, the Insurer should request premium payer representatives, Insurance medical care provider representatives, and experts to study and promote the global budget paymentsystem.

The agenda for the study process (preceding paragraph) and the list of attendees should be announced 7 days prior to the meeting; the minutes of the meeting should be made public within 10 days after the meeting.

The scope of district, mentioned in Paragraph 2, shall be determined by the Insurer and submitted to the Competent Authority for approval.

Article 62

The contracted medical care institutions shall declare to the Insurer the number of points relating to the medical services provided and expense of associated drugs, based on the Fee Schedule and Reference List for Medical Services and the Reference List for Drugs.

Contracted medical care institutions should declare these medical expenses before the first day of the month following treatment, for up to 6 months. However, postponement for expiry is allowed in case of unavoidable circumstances.

The Insurer shall calculate the value of each point, based on the budget specified in the preceding Article, and the total points of medical services rendered, as reviewed by the Insurer. The Insurer shall pay each contracted medical care institution accordingly.

The drug expenses shall be paid to the contracted medical care institutions after being examined by the Insurer. When expenses exceed the pre-set total drug expense ratio target, the Insurer shall adjust the drug expense payment and the payment schedule for the following year. The amount in excess shall be deducted from the budget for the medical benefit payments for the current season, and adjustments shall be made to the payments for contracted medical care institutions, according to expenditure targets.

Article 63

In order to examine the items, quantity, and quality of the medical services provided by this Insurance's contracted medical care institutions, the Insurer shall appoint medical and pharmaceutical specialists who have relevant clinical or other experience to conduct a review. The review should be based on approved payment. This work should be assigned to a relevant professional agency or group.

The review of medical services (preceding paragraph) shall be performed before, during, and after the matter; the methods used will be sampling or case analysis.

The Competent Authority shall establish the procedure and schedule for medical expense application and payment, as well as the rules for reviewing medical services.

The Insurer shall be responsible for drafting the contract items of Paragraph 1, the contracted institutions, qualifications of the group, selection and revision of procedure, supervision, and relevant matters pertaining to rights and responsibilities. The Insurer shall report these matters to the Competent Authority for approval.

Article 64

In cases where other contracted medical care institutions fill prescriptions or conduct lab tests or diagnostic examinations in accordance with a physician's instructions, but the Insurer determines, after the examination, not to pay the benefit because of improper instructions by the physician, the expenses thereof shall be borne by the medical institution where the physician practices, by applying for a reduction of medical expenses.

Article 65

Paragraph 3 of Article 61 and Paragraph 4 of Article 62 may be implemented in stages, with the respective implementation dates being set by the Competent Authority. Before the implementation date, the amount of payment for each point in the Fee Schedule and Reference List for Medical Services shall be decided by the Competent Authority.

Chapter 7 Contracted Medical Care Institutions

Article 66

Medical care institutions should apply to the Insurer to become contracted medical care institutions. The Competent Authority shall determine the qualifications, procedure, review standards, disqualification, resolution of violations, and other relevant matters pertaining to contracted medical care institutions.The medical care institutions of the preceding paragraph are limited to those in Taiwan, Penghu, Kinmen, and Matsu.

Article 67

The provision of wards in a contracted hospital shall comply with the criteria for establishment of an Insurance ward. The criteria for establishment of an Insurance ward, and the ratio of Insurance wards to the aggregate number of hospital wards, shall be established by the Competent Authority.

Contracted hospitals should announce daily the status of their Insurance wards.

The Insurer should announce the ratio of Insurance wards monthly and should conduct quarterly checks.

Article 68

With regard to the medical benefit provided by this Insurance, unless provided otherwise by this Act, the contracted medical care institutions shall not charge beneficiaries for dummy items.

Article 69

The contracted medical care institutions shall check the Insured's qualification when they visit, matching it to the information on their Health Insurance card. The Insurer may refuse to pay medical expenses for those who were not checked, and may seek reimbursement if medical expenses were paid. This is not applicable to matters not attributable to contracted medical care institutions.

Article 70

In the event of an incident to the Insured while they are under coverage, the contracted medical care institution shall provide proper medical service, based on their specialties and facilities, or assist with referral, without any unreasonable refusal due to the status of the Insured.

Article 71

Contracted medical care institutions may give the Insured a prescription after treatment, which may specify dosage, lab tests, and diagnostic examinations.

The Insured's drug prescription, ambulatory treatment, and major lab test items should be stored on the Health Insurance card.

Article 72

To reduce cases of ineffective treatment and other inappropriate uses of medical Insurance resources, the Insurer shall draft an annual proposal for controlling inappropriate use of resources. It shall be presented to the NHIC for discussion, then submitted to the Competent Authority for approval.

Article 73

Contracted medical care institutions that have received medical Insurance payments in excess of a specific amount should present financial reports to the Insurer, signed by a Certified Public Accountant, or reports from an institution that audits National Health Insurance businesses. The Insurer should make this report public.

The Insurer shall draft the rules pertaining to the amounts, deadlines, and procedures for providing financial reports, and the format and content to be presented to the NHIC for discussion and submission to the Competent Authority for approval.

The financial report of Paragraph 1 should include at least the following reports:

1. Asset-liability statement;
2. Surplus balance sheet;
3. Changes in net report;
4. Cash flow report;
5. Medical revenue schedule;
6. Medical cost schedule.

Article 74

The Insurer and the contracted medical care institutions should regularly publicise information pertaining to quality of care of this Insurance.

The Insurer shall draft the scope of quality-of-care information, how it is made public, and other rules pertaining to how it is presented to the NHIC for discussion and later submission to the Competent Authority for approval.

Article 75

When drug expenses applied for by contracted medical care institutions exceed the amount designated by the Competent Authority, contracts for all transactions with pharmaceutical firms should be prepared and signed, to define rights and responsibilities, except where the drugs are purchased for rare diseases or other special cases.

The Competent Authority should meet with the Fair Trade Commission of the Executive Yuan to draft a definitive format for the written contract of the preceding paragraph, and to discuss other recorded or unrecorded matters.

Chapter 8 Reserve Fund and Administrative Expenses

Article 76

In order to balance its finances, this Insurance shall set aside a reserve fund from the following sources:

1. Surplus from each fiscal year;
2. Overdue premium charges for this Insurance;
3. Profits generated from the management of the reserve fund;
4. Social health and welfare surcharge on tobacco and alcohol products, imposed by the Government;
5. Income from sources with statutory grounds other than this Act.

Any deficiency in the balance between Insurance revenue and expenditure for each fiscal year shall be first recovered from the reserve fund.

Article 77

The funds of this Insurance may be managed in the following ways:

1. Investing in treasury bonds, treasury bills, and corporate bonds;
2. Depositing in Government-owned banks or financial institutions designated by the Competent Authority;
3. Investing in any other programme that is beneficial to this Insurance, as approved by the Competent Authority.

Article 78

In principle, the aggregate amount of the reserve fund shall be equal to the aggregate amount of benefit payments in the most recent 1 to 3 months, based on actuarial principles.

Chapter 9 Collecting and Gathering of Relevant Information and Documents

Article 79

The Insurer may require relevant agencies to provide the information it needs to carry out the business of the Insurance. The agencies may not refuse to do so.

The information obtained by the Insurer in accordance with the preceding paragraph should be handled responsibly and prudently. The storage and use of relevant information should be carried out in accordance with the Personal Information Protection Act.

Article 80

In order to review Insurance disputes, or for administrative reasons, the Competent Authority may ask the Insured, the Group Insurance Applicants, the Premium Withholders, and contracted medical care institutions to provide it with relevant documents, such as accounting records, receipts, medical history, diagnosis records, medical expenses, and other documents or relevant information. The Insured, Group Insurance Applicants, Premium Withholders, and contracted medical care institutions shall not elude, reject, obstruct, misrepresent, misreport or misstate the facts.

The Competent Authority shall determine the scope, accessing procedure, and rules for interview and inquiry pertaining to the relevant information.

Chapter 10 Penal Provisions

Article 81

Any person who applies for reimbursements or claims medical expenses through improper conduct, or makes a false certification or report, or a misrepresentation shall be fined a sum the equivalent to 2–20 times the benefits or medical expenses received. If a criminal offence is involved, the person shall also be referred to the Court. Any medical expenses received by a contracted medical care institution may be deducted from the expenses claimed by it.

If the conduct of a Contracted Medical Institution is improper, the Insurer may announce the name of the institution, the responsible medical personnel, and/or the name of the individual and the nature of the violation, depending on the severity of the situation.

Article 82

Any person who violates the provisions of Article 68 shall return the amount received and shall be fined a sum of five times the expenses received.

Article 83

If a contracted medical care institution violates Article 68, or acts as described in Paragraph 1 of Article 81, the Insurer must study the severity of the situation and decide whether to suspend the contract indefinitely or for a period of time.

Article 84

If a Group Insurance Applicant fails to carry out subscription to this Insurance pursuant to Article 15, for the Insured or their dependents, it shall be fined a sum equivalent to 2–4 times the amount of the payable premiums, in addition to the unpaid premium.

The preceding paragraph is not applicable if the failure is not attributable to the Group Insurance Applicant.

If a Group Insurance Applicant fails to pay the premiums for the Insured and his/her dependents, but the premiums were paid by the Insured, the Group Insurance Applicant shall return the premiums paid, and shall be fined a sum equivalent to 2–4 times the amount of the payable premiums.

Article 85

If the Premium Withholder does not deduct the supplementary premium from the Insured, as specified in Article 31, the Insurer shall impose a deadline for making the payment and a fine that is twice the deducted amount. Those who do not pay within the specified deadline shall be fined three times the deducted amount.

Article 86

If the contracted hospital fails to attain the criteria and the specified ratio of Insurance wards, as provided in Article 67, it shall be fined no less than 10,000 and no more than 50,000 New Taiwan Dollars, based on the inadequate number of beds, and shall be ordered to improve within a given period of time. The Insurer should make improvements within the specified time; the fine shall be continuously imposed for each violation, if improvements are not made within the given time.

Article 87

Contracted medical care institutions that violate Paragraph 1 of Article 75, do not sign contracts, or that violate the rules set by the Competent Authority, according to Paragraph 2 of Article 75, regarding what and what not to record, shall be fined not less than 20,000 and not more than 100,000 New Taiwan Dollars. Improvements should be made by the Insurer within the specified time; the fine shall be continuously imposed for each violation if improvements are not made within the given time.

Article 88

If a beneficiary subscribes to this Insurance in violation of the provision of Article 11, they shall be subject to a penalty of no less than 3000 and no more than 15,000 New Taiwan Dollars in addition to payment of the premium shortfall.

The payment of the premium shortfall described in the preceding paragraph is limited to premiums payable within the most recent 5 years.

Article 89

In any of the following cases, a fine of two to four times the amount of the payment of a different premium shall be imposed in addition to the payment of a premium differential:

1. The Insured payroll-related amount of the Insured in Category 1, as declared by the Group Insurance Applicants for the Insured, is less than the regulated Insured payroll-related amount;
2. The Insured payroll-related amount of the Insured in Categories 2 and 3, as declared by the Insured, is less than the regulated Insured payroll-related amount.

Article 90

Any person who violates the provisions of Article 70 or Paragraph 1 of Article 80 shall be subject to a fine of no less than 20,000 and no more than 100,000 New Taiwan Dollars.

Article 91

If a beneficiary violates the provisions of this Act by not subscribing to this Insurance, they shall be subject to a fine of not less than 3000 and not more 15,000 New Taiwan Dollars. The beneficiary shall subscribe to this Insurance retroactively from the date on which they qualified for it. Their benefits shall be suspended until the fine and premium are both fully paid.

Article 92

The fines prescribed in this Act shall be imposed by the Insurer.

Chapter 11 Supplementary Provisions

Article 93

The Insurer may apply to the Court for the provisional seizure of assets, and may be exempted from providing a guarantee to Group Insurance Applicants, Insured persons, or contracted medical care institutions that owe the Insurer relevant payments, or are hiding or transferring assets or avoiding resolving matters.

Article 94

For Insured persons who are covered by occupational injury insurance, the medical expenses incurred from the occupational injury contingency shall be paid by the occupational injury insurance.

The Insurer shall be tasked by the Insurer of Labour Insurance to provide medical benefits for occupational injury insurance.

The Competent Authority shall determine the scope, payment compensation, and other relevant regulations of assistance packages, and meet with the Central Labour Competent Authority for approval.

Article 95

If the Insurer has paid Insurance benefits to a beneficiary for a traffic accident, the Insurer may claim against the Insurer of Compulsory Automobile Liability Insurance to recover the benefits paid.

If a beneficiary makes an indemnity claim against a third party, which arises from an incident covered by this Insurance, the Insurer of this Insurance may, after paying Insurance benefits to the beneficiary, exercise the right of subrogation in accordance with the following subparagraphs:

1. Public safety incidents: the Insurer shall claim against the Insurer of the liability Insurance carried by the third party, as required by the laws and regulations. However, if the indemnity amount is deficient in settlement, the Insurer may claim against the third party for the deficit amount.
2. Other serious traffic accidents, public nuisance, or food poisoning incidents: when the third party has liability Insurance, the Insurer shall claim against the third party's Insurer. If there is any deficit in settlement, or no such Insurance is carried, the Insurer shall claim against the third party for the deficit amount or for the indemnity.

The regulations governing the minimum compensation amount, compensation scope, methods, and procedures for public safety incidents, serious traffic accidents, and public nuisance or food poisoning incidents that are referred to in the preceding paragraph shall be prescribed by the Competent Authority.

Article 96

The revenues and expenditures of this Insurance shall be administered by the Insurer as an Operation Fund in the annual fiscal budget.

Article 97

All account records, receipts, revenue, and expenditure under this Insurance shall be exempted from taxation.

Article 98

The overdue charge, the temporary suspension of benefits, and the fines specified in Article 35, Article 37, Paragraph 2 of Article 50, and Article 91 are not applicable to those Insured who qualify as being in financial difficulty.

Article 99

The Competent Authority may develop a budget to establish a fund for those Insured who have financial difficulty in paying premiums; they may apply for interest-free loans to the amount of the premiums and fees owing under this Insurance.

The monthly repayment may not be higher than two times the personal premium that was set at the time of applying for the loan, unless the borrower wishes to repay it earlier.

The Competent Authority shall determine the loan application, conditions, loan repayment schedule and methods, and other relevant matters of the Reserve Fund of this Insurance.

Article 100

The standards for financial difficulties, defined in the two previous articles, shall be interpreted by the Competent Authority with reference to relevant standards for social subsidies.

Article 101

The Insurer should check, on a regular basis, the ability to pay of those Insured who have applied for premium payment postponement or loan clearing pursuant to paragraphs 1 and 2 of Article 87 (prior to the Act's amendment on 4 January 2011).

Article 102

All accumulated deficits incurred before the amendment of this Act on 4 January 2011 shall be borne by the Central Competent Authority through annual incremental amounts in the national budget.

Article 103

The Competent Authority shall prepare the Enforcement Rules of this Act.

Article 104

The Executive Yuan shall decide upon the date of implementation of this Act.

Amendments to the articles of this Act shall come into force as of the date of its promulgation, with the exception that the implementation date of Article 11 (amended 29 June 2011) shall be determined by the Executive Yuan.

Index

Printed in the United States
by Baker & Taylor Publisher Services